THE GROOMING OF A CHANCELLOR

THE GROOMING
of a
CHANCELLOR

George Alleyne

The University of the West Indies Press
Jamaica • Barbados • Trinidad and Tobago

The University of the West Indies Press
7A Gibraltar Hall Road, Mona
Kingston 7, Jamaica
www.uwipress.com

© 2018 George Alleyne
All rights reserved. Published 2018

A catalogue record of this book is available from the
National Library of Jamaica.

ISBN: 978-976-640-651-6 (print)
       978-976-640-652-3 (Kindle)
       978-976-640-653-0 (ePub)

Cover image: Portrait of Chancellor George Alleyne by David Skinner (2006), UWI Regional Headquarters, Mona, Jamaica.
Cover and book design by Robert Harris
Set in Sabon 10.25/15 x 24

The University of the West Indies Press has no responsibility for the persistence or accuracy of URLs for external or third-party Internet websites referred to in this publication and does not guarantee that any content on such websites is, or will remain, accurate or appropriate.

Printed in the United States of America

*This book is dedicated to my wife, Sylvan,
and our three children, Carol, Andrew and Adrian,
with gratitude for their love and support over the years.*

Contents

Foreword *Julio Frenk* / ix

Preface / xiii

Acknowledgements / xvii

1. Beginnings: The Early Years / 1
2. Growing up in Jamaica and Becoming West Indian: The University College of the West Indies / 19
3. The Postgraduate Years: Internship / 42
4. My Scientific Career: Sojourn from Clinical Medicine / 62
5. The Professor of Medicine: My Appointment / 80
6. The Beginning of the International Odyssey: Leaving Jamaica / 93
7. Reaching the Top: Election as Director of the Pan American Health Organization / 116
8. The Office of Director: Assumption of Office / 133
9. A New International Challenge: The Director General of the World Health Organization / 150
10. A Second Term as Director / 163
11. The Myth of Retirement / 184

Contents

12. The Return of the Pelican: Back at the University of the West Indies / 206

Epilogue / 224

Appendix 1: Lectures and Formal Presentations / 231

Appendix 2: The University of the West Indies Graduation Addresses / 248

Notes / 251

Bibliography / 257

Index / 259

Foreword

Human beings have always expected inspiring words of wisdom from their leaders. These words may come as part of a political speech, a moral exhortation or a literary essay. Sometimes they arrive in the guise of a memoir. This is the case in *The Grooming of a Chancellor*, a judicious account of a fruitful life that is being published, auspiciously, at a time imbued with uncertainty. One of the early definitions of the word *memorie* (the Anglo-French origin of *memoir*) is "something written to be kept in mind".[1] It is the ultimate expression of a personal struggle against oblivion. In its sagest form it is not a struggle against forgetting in general, but against forgetting what is considered to be commendable, admirable or worthy. This is what seems to worry Sir George Alleyne the most. This apprehension is understandable given the fact that Sir George grew up in a culture and a time in which you had to earn the right to draft a memoir.[2]

So with such a humble hesitation starts a recount of a fascinating life story that spreads over two centuries. It begins in St Philip, Barbados, in the early 1930s; continues in of the University of West Indies in the 1960s; acquires an international character in the 1980s and 1990s, crowning a peak in 1995 at the Pan American Health Organization (PAHO); and concludes with the arrival to the chancellery of the University of West Indies just a few years ago.

During his years as a medical student, Sir George was marked by contrasting experiences: on the one hand, the introduction of penicillin, the new miracle antibiotic, and on the other, the shattering effects of a poliomyelitis epidemic that struck Jamaica in 1954. He also witnessed, enthusiastically, the creation of the West Indies Federation – and the failed attempt to create a single unified independent state in the British-controlled

Foreword

Caribbean region – and, eventually, the independence of Jamaica in 1962. He was also fortunate enough to travel to New York at the beginning of the civil rights struggle. There he was instantaneously attracted to and absorbed by the literature of the Harlem Renaissance and the jazz scene, and attended live performances of Louis Armstrong, Dave Brubeck and Oscar Peterson. After graduating from medical school, Sir George worked at the Barbados General Hospital and at the University College London, and then joined the Tropical Metabolism Research Unit of the University of West Indies, a centre established to study infant malnutrition. There he became the pupil of Professor John C. Waterlow and a skilled scientist in the field of clinical nutrition. As a researcher, he was trained to identify a relevant problem, lay out hypotheses, collect information, analyse data and reach reasonable conclusions. And he was taught to do so without allowance or indulgence, as he narrates in a moving speech that he delivered in London to pay tribute to his mentor.[3] The level of excellence achieved by Sir George through rigorous and methodic research would remain present in all of his following endeavours, first as a professor of medicine at the University of West Indies and then as an international civil servant at the Washington, DC, office of PAHO. There he was appointed head of the Research Coordination Unit and then director of the Area of Health Programs, where he helped to change the nature and scope of the regional immunization programme. In collaboration with the renowned Brazilian epidemiologist Ciro de Quadros, and probably inspired by his early experience as a student in Jamaica, he designed an ambitious programme for the eradication of polio from the Americas, which was remarkably successful as the first region in the world to wipe out this devastating disease. Of notable importance to those interested in the politics of global health are Sir George's reflections on his quest to become assistant director and, especially, director of PAHO: his strong bond with his predecessor, the Brazilian physician Carlyle Guerra de Macedo; the then uneasy relationship between PAHO and the Caribbean nations; the critical role that the fifteen countries of the Caribbean Community (CARICOM) play in the election of PAHO's leadership; and the way he dealt with his opponents and their governments.

Even more insightful are his thoughts on the 1997 election of the director general of the World Health Organization (WHO), in which he was a contender. He describes in detail the way he gathered support from the governments of the CARICOM; the huge disparities in the resources available for his campaign versus the resources mobilized by several of his competitors; the content of his campaign, based on his managerial skills; and his disappointment when he acknowledges the geopolitical nature of the process. The most important objection that Sir George makes to the election process of the leading positions at UN agencies refers to secret balloting. He finds out that the process is corruptible when he is approached by one African delegate asking for money for his vote and that of another colleague. And he concludes: "I was then even more persuaded that the system will continue to be open to corruption until there is open voting which will make it clear how every country has voted." After losing the WHO election, Sir George takes this setback – his first in a major contest in his entire life – with equanimity and grace, repeating to himself the following two days this famous quote from Rudyard Kipling: "If you can meet with Triumph and Disaster / and treat those imposters just the same . . ." Back in Washington, DC, he runs, unopposed, for a second term as director of PAHO, pushes even further the notion of equity in health and pan-Americanism, and works hard to consolidate the relationship with the two leading development banks in the region (the World Bank and the Inter-American Development Bank) and to define what he called the "essential functions of public health": "the functions that the state should discharge if the public's health was to be promoted and avoidable illness prevented". In 2003, after being elected director emeritus, he completes his second term as director of PAHO.

The last chapter of this extraordinary memoir deals with his return to his alma mater. Sir George is the first graduate of the University of the West Indies to be appointed chancellor. And far from assuming his new position as a prelude to his retirement, he involves himself in a major transformation of its governance structure, which, among other things, led to the doubling of student enrolment over ten years. In reading Sir George's memoir, one realizes that in addition to excellence, the practice of research and medicine helped him develop the gift of elegance, which he displayed in his various positions. This gift is also present in the recount of his public life, which is tidy and eloquent. He chooses with great tact the relevant moments of his career and discusses them with good judgement and depth. His doubts about the transcendence of writing about what he experienced may well be left behind. He has a good story to tell and a rich perspective derived from a life that includes outstanding experiences in basic science, clinical medicine, global health and higher education. This memoir from a remarkable leader will nourish and inspire the lives of those seeking to make our world a better place. His basic lesson is particularly timely: the need to strive for what is true and what is just.

Julio Frenk, MD, PhD
President of the University of Miami and former Minister of Health of Mexico

NOTES

1. "Memoir", Dictionary.com, http://www.dictionary.com/browse/memoir. Accessed 28 February 2017.
2. N. Genzlinger, "The Problem with Memoirs", *New York Times*, 30 January 2011. http://www.nytimes.com/2011/01/30/books/review/Genzlinger-t.html?pagewanted=all&_r=0. Accessed 28 February 2017.
3. G. Alleyne, "The Houses That John Built", http://wphna.org/wp-content/uploads/2014/12/1996-George-Alleyne-on-JCW.pdf. Accessed 7 March 2017.

Preface

Colleagues and friends kept asking, "When will you write?" or saying more insistently, "You *must* write." I was finally convinced by those many persons for whom I have respect and affection that the story of a boy from rural Barbados who travelled far and wide, interacted with some of the world's leaders, and played a significant role in major regional and international institutions was worth sharing. In telling the story now, I have relived, sometimes with considerable excitement, the journey, and the episodes and relationships that have formed me.

Unfortunately, I had not been so convinced from my earliest days that I would be of some historical importance that I kept records of all I did or said. As a young man, I looked askance at those who kept diaries or records as bordering on the narcissistic or arrogant. Perhaps I have been influenced by one of my early, very charismatic teachers – Professor Norman Millott, professor of zoology. He would often refer to his lectures as elucidating points that were not found in textbooks, but when he was asked why he did not write a textbook, his response was, "Only second-rate chaps write books."

For two reasons, there are few pictures of my early years. The first is that a camera was a luxury we could not afford, and the second is that our family moved so often that many records were lost along the way.

On taking the decision to write, I had to choose whether to produce a memoir that depended heavily on archival research and documentation to substantiate the many judgements I had made and decisions I had taken. I decided that I had neither the time nor temperament for such an approach. Perhaps I am swayed by my visceral aversion to historical determinism, but more important, I did not believe this would make for interesting reading.

Preface

There are enough Caribbean historians, and if there are not enough now to chronicle the events that surround my life, surely there will be future PhD students to fill these gaps. I decided on a more personal account of my life and times, going beyond mere stories, and referring to sources and references only when necessary.

This work is roughly chronological. The first part covers my early upbringing and schooling. These were years in which my native Barbados was awakening from its colonial past and passing through the same social unrest and upheaval experienced throughout the Caribbean. I was a bright boy, but still a boy, when I left home at age nineteen and entered upon the next major and formative part of my life. That was spent in Jamaica in the fledgling University College of the West Indies, from which I graduated in medicine. I describe the rationale for my choosing what to many of my parents' friends and advisers represented an uncertain academic future. But it was in the university and Jamaica that I became a West Indian man. I learned to manage my time and balance competing social and academic interests and responsibilities. And it was in Jamaica, too, that I found my wife, or perhaps she found me.

Then came my further training in academic medicine, my exhilarating days in research, where success often depended on overcoming the challenges inherent in the status of developing world institutions. I entered the world of international health timidly at first, but soon I acquired the professional and political skills necessary for success. When I retired formally from that sphere, I continued to be engaged in health in the Caribbean and globally, emphasizing even more forcibly the role of health in national development. In the many tributes paid to me in recent years, the role of helping to promote the wider place of health has garnered most encomiums. And then I returned emotionally if not physically to the university, which I regard as my Capistrano in the Caribbean. I regard much of my previous life and experience as the grooming I needed for the position of chancellor, which I held for fourteen years.

Health in its many and varied dimensions is the theme that has dominated my professional life. At first it was the health of individuals – learning the healing craft. Then it was a search for those factors that perturb equilibrium and lead to disease. I then taught elements of the craft, expanding the horizons of the young beyond the curative to embrace the social as well, and by example teaching them how to help patients deal with death and recognize the ineffable tragedy of the human condition. From there I moved on to meld my technical with managerial skills and play a major role in health policies requiring international action. In this phase, I would argue and write about health as instrumental for human development, and cooperation in health as crucial for the Caribbean.

Perhaps one important purpose of a memoir such as this is to transmit to one's grandchildren something of one's life and times and provide another tie that might bind them together. And I can hold up many mentors and give credit to many relationships and individuals critical to this journey, but there are none more important than my wife Sylvan, to whom I dedicate this memoir.

But enough of procrastination! In Churchill's words, "Come then, let us to the task!"

Acknowledgements

Many of the persons responsible for my academic and professional development have been mentioned at appropriate places throughout the text. Here I wish to thank mainly those who stimulated and helped me to record the more important incidents of the journey which took me from Barbados to Jamaica to Washington, DC, and points beyond. They inspired me to think of that journey as grooming me to be chancellor of the University of the West Indies.

I am enormously grateful to my wife, Sylvan; my siblings; those former students who have been persistent over the years in insisting that I should write this; and Valerie Facey and Bridget Brereton who also urged me along. I wish to thanks especially my sister Jacqueline, who not only encouraged me at the appropriate moments but read and critiqued some of the earlier versions of the manuscript. I thank Julio Frenk for having agreed to write the foreword and this is yet another indication of his support to me over many years. I have a deep appreciation for the encouragement and support of the University of the West Indies Press, especially chair Luz Longsworth and general manager Joseph Powell, but special thanks and gratitude go to my editor Shivaun Hearne for her patient, expert guidance during the process. Her careful editing and apt suggestions for change improved the manuscript enormously. I also wish to thank Allyson Latta, my development editor for her input. My able assistant Silvia Sanchez has been invaluable throughout – keeping track of the manuscript, copying photographs, researching material and paying attention to the many important details that had to be taken care of. I also acknowledge the many colleagues, particularly in the University of the West Indies and the Pan American Health Organization, who directly or indirectly supplied me

Acknowledgements

with information and whose support has contributed not only to the book but to the journey itself. Finally, I wish to thank the Pan American Health Organization and the current director, Dr Carissa Etienne, for providing the facilities I needed for this work.

CHAPTER 1

Beginnings
The Early Years

There is a Jamaican proverb which says "Yam don't grow potato", indicating that one is a product of one's forebears. I must therefore set all that has occurred in my life against theirs and begin by sharing something about my parents. My father, Clinton Ogarren Alleyne, born 20 June 1907, was the last child of Wilhemina and Joseph Alleyne, who lived all their lives in Merricks, a small village in St Philip, Barbados, near to the sea. I heard stories of a brother who drowned at the neighbouring beach, and my Uncle Fitz had acquired the name of "burnt boy", because as a child he was burnt by a kitchen fire and still bore the scars in his face. It was said that he was saved because he was wrapped in plantain leaves until his skin healed. Two sisters, Brontilla and Ethel, migrated to the United States, and one brother, Charles, to Trinidad and Tobago, where he became a distinguished reporter for the *Trinidad Guardian* newspaper.

My father attended Holy Trinity Boys School, and after finishing the seventh standard, he became first a pupil teacher and then took and passed the necessary exams to be a qualified teacher. From all accounts, this was his natural calling, and he excelled at it. He studied for an intermediate bachelor of arts degree from London University through correspondence courses, but he never did take the examination. He taught at Holy Trinity, which was one of the many schools established by the Anglican Church in Barbados. Church ownership was made clear when the priest of the church, Reverend Brandt, would come to school at the end of the month with a little black satchel, summon the teachers to the platform and pay them in cash in front of the whole school.

I had the impression that my father was the de facto deputy headmaster. He was the Scouts master, he organized the school garden, the produce from which won many prizes at the annual agricultural exhibition, and he was a respected member of the local community. Many came to him for advice and often brought their children to be disciplined. He read voraciously and was a physical fitness fanatic. He died at the early age of forty-five of chronic renal failure, and I still regret that I do not have my mother's letters describing his hospital stay, the hope she had for his recovery, the days around his death and his funeral. There she was, a young widow at age forty-two, with two children at university and five young ones at home, and no immediate source of support. My sister Cynthia and I decided not to return home from Jamaica for his funeral, as we believed that the money for our fares was better spent in supporting the family.

My mother, Eileen Allanmoore (née Gaskin), was born 22 September 1911, and grew up in East Point in St Philip with her aunt and cousins, as her mother had emigrated to New York. I heard little of my grandfather except that he had gone to Panama to work on the canal, and then to Brazil, where he died of some diarrheal illness working on the railroad. Like many lower-middle-class girls whose families could not afford the fees for post-primary education, my mother attended the local equivalent of a finishing school at a stern dowager's home, where she learned to sew, crochet, play the piano, sing and be instructed in manners befitting a lady. She was a member of various church groups – choir, altar guild, and so on. At age twenty, she married my father and dedicated herself to homemaking and, as time went on, raising a family of seven. In spite of meagre domestic resources, which she supplemented with activities such as baking and sewing (in which she was assisted by sundry young women who were apprenticed to her), she delighted in entertaining. She was a great conversationalist, had a remarkable way with words, was a lover of books and frequently played the role of domestic counsellor to both men and women in days when domestic violence was not uncommon.

After my father died, she had to find gainful occupation, so she became the parish librarian, and many successful Barbadian men and women from the area recount her bringing them into the library and introducing them to the pleasures of books. She had her first stroke at about age fifty and her second about ten years later. She never recovered from the second one and spent the last four or five years in a chronic-care hospital, aphasic and with a dense hemiparesis. In later years, as I learned more about cerebral function and cognition, I have been horrified at the thought of her being conscious of her inability to speak, all the while trapped in a wordless nightmare.

I was born on 7 October 1932 in Lucas Street, St Philip, Barbados. I am the first child of that marriage which produced seven children, and I do think I had a special place in my mother's affection, as she was pregnant at the time she married, and in those days to have a child out of wedlock was an egregious sin. For many years, in our church, children who were born to single mothers were baptized on Wednesdays, while those born to married couples were baptized on Sundays. My coming meant that she put on hold other plans for her personal development. From all accounts I was a healthy baby, breast-fed and supplemented with Cow and Gate infant formula. I write this mischievously, because as a public health advocate, I too have railed against the infamy of Nestlé in selling infant formula to poor mothers.

For five years, we lived in Lucas Street in a small four-room wattle-and-daub house, and I have vivid recollections of our home, its surroundings, and the presence of almond and sweet apple trees in our yard. I recall my mother dusting the green apples with flour, which she thought would deter the schoolboys from picking them, just in case the white stuff was not flour. My siblings greet with sceptical derision my claim that I remember being placed in my crib in the shade of a breadfruit tree at about six months of age. The life and status of schoolteacher required that we have a maid, although for the life of me I cannot imagine how my parents would have employed one on my father's meagre salary.

But perhaps the first formative event of my life was one that occurred before I was five years old, when I accompanied my father to Holy Trinity Elementary School, where he taught. I had learned to read at about age four, and according to my mother, I was fascinated by and had a reverence for books at a very early age. And even then, I had ambitions. One day I saw a fife and drum band of young boys in smart khaki uniforms marching to the neighbouring King George V Memorial Park for some celebration and said to my mother that I so wished to be part of a similar band. She dissuaded me, explaining that the band was from a reform school not too far away, and perhaps my ambition might be channelled in other directions.

Another formative experience was the warmth of family gatherings, which instilled in me an appreciation of the value of the family. My grandmother lived in Merricks village, about five miles away, and I have vivid memories of gatherings at her house at the end of the year, when our family, my uncle and his family, and sundry cousins would congregate to eat, drink and make speeches. There was lots of delicious cake, and bags of stored peanuts. If one made a small hole in the bag, one could eat enough to get sick, which I did on one occasion. When we crawled under the house to the cellar, we discovered piles of yams stored in ashes and empty bottles with marbles inside. I presume the latter were the equivalent of soda bottles, and the marbles were stoppers. I was amazed at the ingenuity of the manufacturers in getting marbles into bottles, when I could not get them out. But what has remained with me, in recalling these gatherings, is an indissoluble bond between members of our family.

After five years in Lucas Street, we moved to Merricks village to be near my grandmother, whom I remember as a kindly old lady who thought nothing of trying to discipline my father physically even when he was age thirty-two, for what I recall was some minor infraction such as not being sufficiently respectful to her. Her death was heralded by cooing doves and howling dogs. Family lore says that when she died at the ripe old age of seventy-six, her mother, Grand Nan, who lived to be 106 and called my grandmother "Babe", on learning of her death was heard to say, "I knew I would never raise that child. She was always sickly."

The 1930s were a period of intense political turmoil and struggle, and the social conditions in Barbados were among the worst in the West Indies. The unrest culminated in the 1937 riots, which were confusing and traumatic to a five-year-old, and I was led to understand that they represented attempts to overthrow the established British colonial order. That system had engendered a level of social injustice which was not immediately obvious to me, as it was the order of the day, but I do remember feeling anxiety and fear at seeing the shop next door broken into and ransacked during the riots, and seeing the young men of the village hunted by black policeman with long guns and arrested for taking the barest of material necessities from shops in the village. Because of the general unrest, my father actually bought a gun, much to my mother's consternation, although I don't think he ever used it.

Life as a schoolboy in Merricks seemed to comprise just two periods – school and vacation. I now walked to Holy Trinity School, all three miles twice daily. Although my father taught in the school and rode his bicycle there, he would never take me. On occasion he would pass me on the road with the comment, "You are late." Of course, punishment went with being late, and many were the days when I would take shortcuts and run across a cane field to beat the bell that marked the beginning of class. I suppose it was on the days I did not make it that my attention to punctuality was, perhaps literally, imprinted on me.

The start of the school term was always a miserable affair, as children were dosed with castor oil to rid them of the toxins that had accumulated from the fruits and foods of dubious cleanliness they consumed during vacation and any worms that might inhibit their learning. At this time I learned to be impressed by folk medicine; the elders knew the various bushes that could be boiled into teas or made into poultices to cure the numerous ailments from which we were afflicted. Luckily in my case, ethnomedicine, one of the practices left from slavery, had no deleterious effects.

WE WERE SEVEN

I am still amazed that seven of us survived to adulthood, as we were born into a Barbados which had some of the worst social conditions in the Caribbean. Infant mortality was high, and I had only a thirty per cent chance of seeing my first birthday. I often reflect that Clinton and Eileen would not have been displeased with how we turned out.

My sister Cynthia was born in Lucas Street in 1934. After high school, she entered the University College of the West Indies on a Government Exhibition, and after graduating, gaining a teaching diploma and teaching in a Jamaican school, she went off to France, where she married her childhood sweetheart, Ronald, who had become a surgeon. They then moved to Morocco, where he practised. She returned to Barbados to join the Foreign Service, but even then, and more so after retirement, she dedicated most of her time and energy to the arts and culture. She is a prolific writer, and I was so pleased to see her receive recently the Companion of Honour for distinguished national achievement and the inaugural Imagination Award for her contribution to the arts.

Grant was born in Merricks in 1938 and was always something of an enigma to the rest of us. He is no longer with us, but the memory of him and his passing never seems to fade. Immediately after his birth, the skies opened, and it rained almost continuously for six weeks. Cynthia, who was then four years old, was confident that the stork which brought him had left a hole in the sky through which the water was pouring. Hot water seemed to be all-important around the birth of young children, as it was needed to attend to the mother, who would stay in bed for nine days after the birth and to bathe the baby and wash the diapers. We had no hot water because there was no dry wood around to make a fire. My father had to cut down a fence of what we knew as "moabite", which burned when green, and thus make a fire to boil the water.

Grant's childhood and elementary school days were unremarkable, as I recall. He attended St Margaret's and St Martin's elementary schools and at age twelve went off to Harrison College. But by the time I was leaving for university, my mother was already lamenting his poor performance in school, part of which I have always believed was due to his being compared with his older siblings. There was a dramatic change when my father died, however, and Grant began to dedicate himself seriously to school and study. On leaving school, he taught briefly and then entered the government civil service, took and passed, by external study, a bachelor of arts degree from London University. This was no mean achievement. He married Sybil Maxwell, the daughter of one of my father's old teaching contemporaries, and had a son, George.

He then decided to study medicine, came to Jamaica with his family and lived with us for several years. After graduating and completing an internship, he went to the United States and entered a residency training programme in obstetrics and gynaecology. His residency completed and specialist examinations passed, he moved to Fayetteville in North Carolina, to establish a successful practice. Apparently he was the first black obstetrician/gynaecologist in that town. We corresponded fitfully, and I heard news of his professional and personal progress. Becoming enamoured of finance, he dedicated himself seriously to studying the American financial system, and he did very well indeed from his investments.

His first major tragedy was the death of his son, George, who was outstanding academically. As Grant told it, he was in his office one morning in April 1983, when Sybil, who worked in his office, received a telephone call from Brown University. George, a freshman who was fulfilling the brilliant promise he had shown as a student up to that time, had been found dead in his room. He had told his mother a few days before that he was suffering from a viral respiratory infection, and the postmortem showed that he died of heart failure from a viral myocarditis.

As Grant would describe it later, his whole world came crashing down, as his hopes had been for George to qualify as a physician and take over his practice or establish a similar one of his own. His daughter, Sylvia, was not as intellectually gifted as George. Grant and I became closer after George's death, corresponding often by telephone, and he would go on to be an outstanding presence at the weddings of our three children – tall, with a greying beard, a loud voice, and an incredible memory. He could recite long passages of poetry he had learned in elementary school. He remembered all the verses of Macaulay's *Lays of Ancient Rome* and would have no hesitation in reciting them.

Then one day in June 2005, he called to say that he wished to come to Washington, because he wanted to see my internist. He had a medical problem and was seeking another opinion. He had been suffering from diabetes for some time, had been self-medicating, and now had a severe infection of his foot. I advised that he obtain a medical opinion first so that I could have the information to pass to my internist. He went to the emergency room at the local hospital and was immediately admitted; his diabetes was uncontrolled, and he had gangrene of his right lower leg.

It was steady deterioration from there on. One leg was amputated, then the other, and he developed every possible organ complication of diabetes – gut, heart, brain and his kidneys. Eventually he had to be dialysed because of severe renal failure, became demented because of cerebrovascular involvement, and died after seven years of progressively failing health. Sybil, who was nothing short of angelic in caring for him during those trying years, became ill herself and died three years later.

Leonora, the fourth sibling, was born at Long Bay in 1943, and we say that she arrived in a blaze of glory. I was old enough to appreciate when everything was ready for her birth. The cap and the booties had been knitted, the diapers made, washed and ironed, and the midwife had been properly installed at home. My mother duly went into labour, and at the appropriate moment, my father was sent to the kitchen to boil water, which I had learned by then was essential for the delivery. He pumped the small pressure stove, lit it, and there was mighty whoosh as the whole thing seemed to explode in flames. Much to everyone's horror, my mother leapt from her bed, rushed to the kitchen, pushed aside my hapless father, grasped the flaming stove and threw it through the door into the backyard. Whereupon she hurried back to bed and gave birth. Leonora must have been the only one of us born without the necessary basin of hot water in attendance. After leaving school, she trained as a secretary and became executive secretary to the president of the Caribbean Development Bank before emigrating to Britain and Canada. She retired from the Ontario government civil service as a senior administrator.

Cecily was born in Martins Bay in 1946 and also trained as a secretary. She followed Leonora to the Caribbean Development Bank, from which she retired as a senior secretary.

Jacqueline was born in Martins Bay two years later. She won a Barbados Scholarship, graduated from the University of the West Indies and pursued a distinguished career in university administration, eventually becoming registrar of the Cave Hill campus of the university.

Peter was born in St Martins in 1951. Also a graduate of the University of the West Indies, he pursued a career in journalism, but he is perhaps best known in Barbados as Adonijah, a prominent calypsonian.

Beginnings: The Early Years

THE SCHOOL YEARS

After four years at Merricks, we moved to Long Bay, in the same parish, to a house my father built or, rather, paid to have built. He was naturally proud of having bought a quarter of an acre of land and constructing a house, one of whose most attractive features was a broad verandah on three sides, long enough for racing or playing cricket. Those were days of long vacations, and playing as all young boys of that day played – making and flying our kites, playing marbles, and playing cricket with makeshift bats and balls. We read and studied by the light of a kerosene lamp, as there was no electricity. The news was gleaned from the daily newspaper and the Barbados Rediffusion, which was in effect a speaker linked by wire to a central broadcasting station in Bridgetown. The only radio was a couple miles away in King George V Park, where my father would go to listen to broadcasts of boxing and news about the war. Our house was now only about a mile and a half from school, and the routine was much the same as in our previous home. I did well in school and won my first prize for an essay on the donkey, for which I received a copy of Robert Louis Stevenson's *Treasure Island*. Throughout my years in elementary school I learned to appreciate that being the teacher's son brought no privileges, perhaps even the reverse.

I had seen pictures of Christmas trees, and at about age twelve, I decided that we should have one, so I obtained a branch of a Barbadian cherry tree from our neighbour, set it in a bucket of sand, dressed it with balloons and candles and placed the wrapped presents under it. My parents were supportive, and the whole family joined in the fun as the candles were lit and carols sung. There must have been some nervousness on their part at the sight of burning candles on a tree in a corner of a wooden house, but a bucket of water stood by.

My father coached me in after-school lessons to prepare me for a government scholarship. There was one scholarship to the island's major first-grade secondary school – Harrison College – and three or so scholarships to the second-grade secondary schools. Teachers at the various elementary schools vied in the preparation of candidates. Much of the coaching took place in the undercroft of the school. Our school was near the church and its graveyard, and given the shallow nature of Barbadian soil, graves often had to be dug through stone, so we lived with the frequent sound of falling stones from dynamite blasts. Infant mortality was high, and the coffins of young children which passed often before us as we sat in the undercroft were wrapped in mauve cloth. To this day, that colour evokes in me a feeling of sadness.

I took the first-grade exam for the first time in 1943 and placed sixth, much to my father's annoyance, but gained one of the scholarships to a second-grade secondary school, which my father declined. He blamed my failure on the fact that, and I quote him, "You take after your mother – you are a Gaskin." My mother was comforting, noting, of course, that there was nothing wrong in being a Gaskin. The next year I took and won the first-grade scholarship – the first time a boy from St Philip had done so – and my father was pleased, because, after all, according to him I was an Alleyne. My mother held her peace. The scholarship paid tuition plus five pounds per term.

These were Second World War years, when we were fed diets of patriotic songs and collected thin silver paper wrappers from packages of cigarettes for the war effort. There were shortages of almost every material, as well as food. There was a call to be self-reliant and plant vegetables, so one year there was a glut of sweet potatoes throughout the community, and my mother ingeniously prepared them in myriad ways. They were boiled, baked, steamed, grated and mixed with various spices to form savoury meals. We were even introduced to whale meat, which was dubbed "arctic steak".

Schoolboys told tall tales of seeing German submarines and foreign sailors coming ashore at night. The seniors at Holy Trinity circulated a rumour that Reverend Brandt, because of his name, had to be a German spy, and we swore that his radio was in fact a transmitter through which he sent strategic critical messages to Germany about his parish. It was a manifestation of our self-importance and arrogance to believe that the goings and comings of rural folk were of critical importance to German intelligence.

After four years in Long Bay, we moved to Martins Bay, because my father was appointed headmaster of tiny St Margaret's Boys School, in the parish of St John. The appointment apparently depended on the approval of the priest there, and I recall my father being taken by the local priest to visit the one responsible for the school and lobbying various important personages, such as local plantation owners, for the appointment. We lived in a rented house, literally a stone's throw from the beach, and I spent long days on the beach, walking on the shoals as the tide receded to visit caves filled with beautiful sea anemones.

I got to display my entrepreneurial bent in several ways. My mother thought of supplementing the household income by baking and selling cakes, the only drawback being that she had no oven. So I took a wooden case, lined it with tin, and made an oven which she could place on the top of an oil-burning stove. We stopped excessive heat loss by placing a wet crocus bag on top. I also fashioned the necessary baking tins, and for some time she had a small baking business, which I believe faltered eventually because no strict line could be drawn between domestic consumption and production for sale.

One of my father's accomplishments was the merger of the boys' and girls' schools, which caused much consternation in the local community. In Martins Bay, he again became involved in all aspects of community life, and he and my mother were pillars of the small Anglican church. I have pleasant memories of the fishermen – their lives and even their loves – and fish, being made to drink shark's liver oil, and exercising frantically, as I tried unsuccessfully to develop the kind of musculature my father had. I would spend hours next door watching men cut and saw wood to build fishing boats and would listen to the stories of the master builder, Stanley Greaves. Sometimes he would smoke his pipe and mournfully sing a song which I still recall:

> Who will smoke my meerschaum pipe,
> Who will smoke my meerschaum pipe,
> When I am far away?

I doubt he knew what a meerschaum pipe was, but perhaps I underestimate him. As I watched the boats come and go and heard tales of the dangers the fishermen faced, I developed a deep appreciation, as Psalm 107 says, for "they that go down to the sea in ships, that do business in great waters".

My father's final assignment was as headmaster of St Martin's Boys School in St Philip, so we moved to St Martins in 1949. This was a bigger school, and again he and my mother became involved in the church and community activities. The characteristics of which his former pupils speak when I meet them are his punctuality and his being a strict disciplinarian in days when discipline was enforced by the recognition of authority and by corporal punishment.

In St Martins, we reconnected with my aunts Ethel and Brontilda (Bron), who had migrated to New York in the 1930s. Aunt Bron's husband, Simeon, visited Barbados in 1950 after an absence of many years and brought with him a barrel of goodies for us. There were tins of various juices, fruits and cookies which I had never seen, as well as second-hand clothes, some of which I wore gladly. It was my attention to some of his needs that endeared me to him. For example, when he was going to church and his black serge suit was badly rumpled, I offered to clean and press it for him, there being no dry cleaners in our village. I set to work with sponge, newspaper and steam iron, and eventually handed him his smartly cleaned and pressed suit.

In those later teen years, I would try my hand at fixing almost anything, provided I had the necessary tools. When we moved to St Martins, many of the windows in the house assigned to the headmaster were broken, and some walls were peeling, so I learned how to remove old and insert new glass panes, to mix paint and to boil glue. Not all my efforts were equally successful. I plastered the walls of my room with a sand and lime mixture of the wrong proportions, and the hygroscopic nature of the lime meant that the walls were always wet, so they had to be scraped and plastered again with an appropriate cement mixture.

Because there were few distractions in these urban settings, we relied on ourselves and books for entertainment. The presence of books in the house and their importance were notable. On occasion, when my father had conjunctivitis or laryngitis or some other mild illness and was laid up for a couple of days, or when he just simply wished me to do so, I would read to him for hours. He possessed a trunk of books, which I read, although some of them I could not understand, and one that featured graphic pictures of anatomy was read over and over (without his knowledge, of course). I had

Beginnings: The Early Years

read Tolstoy's *Anna Karenina* by age nine, and I still have the book with my father's signature. I had read *Hamlet* and *Henry IV* many times, and *Tom Brown's Schooldays* and the Pollyanna series were standard fare. I read the adventures of W.E. Johns's Biggles and of Richmal Crompton's irrepressible, mischievous schoolboy William, and the whole family read over and over Gene Stratton Porter's *Laddie* and *A Girl of the Limberlost*. My mother would take the bus to Bridgetown perhaps weekly, and one of the most important things she did there was to go to the Carnegie Public Library. I cannot remember any time in my life in which the written word was not important to me. Books were also important to our concept of family, as we all read the same books, and even today my siblings recall certain passages that we all read over and over.

My brothers and sisters are among the best raconteurs I have ever met, and my brother-in-law Eslie has no peer. His recounting of his days growing up in St Philip is the stuff of movies, and he was not to be outdone by my brothers Grant or Peter. I have dined out repeatedly on one of his stories: A young gentleman in the village took some cloth to a tailor to make him a wedding suit, and he was specific in his instructions. He wished a three-piece suit, which even then was commonly accepted as being a jacket, trousers and a vest or waistcoat. The tailor gave firm assurances that he was experienced in fashioning three-piece suits. When the gentleman returned for his suit on the morning of the wedding, he was presented with three pieces – a jacket, trousers and a cloth cap.

Such stories shaped our thinking and even our play. Having read the story of Robin Hood at about eight or nine years of age, I encouraged my sister Cynthia, who was two years younger than I, to enact one of the scenes I had read of Robin and Little John battling while standing on a log – both armed with staves. I had my staff, and my sister hers. According to the script, I would strike, and she, as Little John, was supposed to parry, but my blow to her head was not fully parried. My mother was not amused when she was called because her daughter was unconscious. I should be grateful that that blow had no impact on her intellectual development, although the counterfactual can never be proved.

HARRISON COLLEGE

So off I went to Harrison College in 1944 in my smart khaki uniform, long woollen socks and crested cap, preening myself and thinking that I looked like any proper English schoolboy. And Harrison College did nothing to erase that image of a good English education fitting a boy for anything in life. The college was founded in 1733 as Harrison Free School "for the poor and indigent boys of the parish". When I entered, it was arguably the finest "first-grade" school in Barbados, excelling academically and in sport. The emphasis was on an academic education with little concern for the technical or vocational skills, and the school prided itself as being patterned on an English grammar school, with the classics as the preeminent subjects. The headmasters and many of the masters were British, although during my stay an increasing number of Barbadian masters were appointed. The school reflected the social and cultural elitism of the racially divided Barbadian society and perhaps to some extent was responsible for maintaining it. We were made to feel proud that alumni of Harrison College shone in various academic and other fields in Britain. Ralph Jemmot's *History of Harrison College*[1] sets out in fine detail the origin, development and contribution of the school. My time there was a pleasant one academically, and otherwise filled with escapades every schoolboy encounters. There was a shortage of textbooks, and my entrepreneurial spirit took me to several second-hand bookstores, where I would rummage and occasionally find copies of required texts. I would buy them, investing money given to buy my lunch, repair them with paper and the juice from the berries of a local tree, popularly known as the clammy cherry, and sell them. I frequently turned quite a handsome profit in the transaction.

Public transport became a problem, as the bus did not come to Martins Bay daily. My sister Cynthia, who was attending Queen's College, and I lived during the week with our cousin Vera and came home on weekends. Vera was married to a policeman and lived in Two Mile Hill in St Michael, from where we could walk to school. I remain deeply indebted to Vera and her husband for taking us in and caring for two teenagers in a small house and with modest means. This permitted me to participate in after-school activities such as sports, at which I was never very good, but like many

Beginnings: The Early Years

of my peers, I tried hard and would gain points for my house by reaching certain minimum standards.

I will never forget two schoolmasters who are in part responsible for my subsequent progress. When I was admitted in 1944, I was placed in form 1B. After three weeks, when the master, Rudolph Daniel, noted that I was getting perfect scores in every test, he had me promoted to 1A. That meant I had to learn Latin, in which I was tutored by a family friend, Mr Gittens. At the end of that first term, when I placed first in the class, I was promoted to the second form, where Greek was taught. I then had to be coached in Greek during the holidays by a master, Carlisle Burton. I am eternally grateful to Carlisle Burton and Rudolf Daniel, who recognized my ability. Had I remained in the class to which I was originally assigned and in which I did not have to extend myself, I might have found less socially acceptable ways to expend my mental energy.

Three aspects of my life at Harrison College influenced me significantly. The first was my appreciation of the importance of social class differences even in that setting. Colour in some cases appeared to trump scholastic ability, and as far as I was concerned, there was no social interaction. I had no white friends, and only on the playing fields did there seem to be genuine intercourse.

We black schoolboys were all conscious of the whites-only clubs such as the Royal Barbados Yacht Club and the Aquatic Club, and we were permitted to attend the latter twice per year. Once was for the swimming sports, which were held at the Aquatic Club, as there was no swimming pool at our school. The other was to see a movie of one of Shakespeare's plays. My mother would recount apocryphal stories of black Barbadians who had gone to Britain to study and had married white girls who had been kind to them there. On return to Barbados, the wives could join those clubs, but the husbands could not.

The second influence was the development of an even greater appreciation for books and literature. The Carnegie Public library was my second home. I read avidly – adventure, crime, philosophy, anything – but remained ignorant of things Caribbean. I was fascinated by the ability of a writer to express ideas so well, and I recall vividly, as a sixth former, hearing Cameron Tudor, who had been to Oxford University, mesmerize us with an address to our literary club – the Acton Club, which I suppose was named after the famous English intellectual Lord Acton. Many quotations are attributed to Acton, but the one I always remembered from school is that "the will of the people cannot make just that which is unjust".

The third aspect of life in Harrison College that shaped me was the discipline of study. I agonized many a night over a mathematical problem by the light of the kerosene lamp with the "Home Sweet Home" chimney, and stuck to it, sometimes in tears, until I found the solution. Many were the occasions when in class I was not asked a question or called upon to translate, but I never attended without being prepared. It is easy to underestimate the value of the discipline of high school – of the years twelve to eighteen – but if such discipline does not become second nature by the end of adolescence, it is extremely difficult if not impossible to acquire it or have it inculcated later. Life at university is so different – learning there is self-generated.

Sports were important to me and the majority of my contemporaries, and I tried my best but was really never any good. I did not have binocular vision, as I had a macular scar from being struck in the left eye when I was about ten years old. I always give this as the reason why I did not become a test cricket player. But I did try at cricket and football and duly participated in athletics in order to reach the required standard and gain points for my house. In Walter Mitty fashion, I saw myself as a first-class cricketer and annoyed my mother immensely by saying to her once that given the choice, I would rather play for the school's First Eleven cricket team than win a Barbados Scholarship. To say that she was upset is an understatement.

My love for cricket, which has never waned, was nourished by my frequent interaction with our head groundsman, Joe Frank. I remember him as tall, elegant, with a military bearing, always with a tie and rarely without a grey felt hat. If I came to school early, I would go to his office, which was redolent with the smell of the linseed oil he used to season the cricket bats. Sometimes he would be wrapping string dipped in glue around the ends of bats that showed signs of wear, and he would recount tales of the feats of the schoolboy cricketers he had seen and coached. He was adamant that there were only three secrets to good bowling, fast or slow – they were length, length, length – which indeed has been and will always be the secret of good bowling. Spin, turn, swing are all important, but only effective when superimposed on good length.

I also joined the boxing club and was the best in my weight (148 pounds) in school. But to be honest, there were not that many of us in the club. That fact in no way dimmed the enthusiasm of our master, Rudolph Daniel, who was our coach. But my pugilistic career came to an abrupt end on a Saturday afternoon when I was about sixteen years old, in an interschool competition between Harrison College and the Lodge School another first-grade school located in St John. My opponent at my weight was a bruiser named Boy Perkins. I came out feinting and jabbing in the opening moments of the first round, and then knew no more. We did win the competition, but my most vivid memory is of a headache, the likes of which I had never had before and have rarely had since. When my mother was told of the incident, she quite pithily instructed me to "Stop this damn foolishness", for which advice I have been ever grateful. Given that I only had macular vision in one eye, it was more than foolhardy to box, but I am quick to add to this account the fact that Boy Perkins went on to box professionally and, I think, became the Caribbean welterweight champion.

The vision in my left eye became impaired in this way. It was a Saturday morning sometime in 1943, when I accompanied my father to school to look after the garden for which he was responsible. Some of the schoolboys about my age would take cans of water from the school to the garden, a distance of about one to two hundred yards, as there was no water supply at or close to the garden. As a group of us returned with empty cans, we played at boxing, and a boy named Frank Ward struck me. I went virtually blind in my left eye. After about a week, I was taken to see the ophthalmologist, who diagnosed a haemorrhage and said nothing could be done. Eventually the blood reabsorbed, but I was left with a macular scar, which means that I have only peripheral vision in that eye. One of my siblings once joked that I had done reasonably well in life with good vision from one eye, and perhaps I might have done *really* well with good binocular vision.

I did well in school – coming top or near top of every class through the years, with many prizes to show for it. I read classics in the sixth form – Latin, Greek, ancient history and literature. The sixth form had two levels –the lower and upper forms. The giants of the upper classical sixth sat in order of length of stay in the form, with the elders at the end of the row. One student actually stayed in the sixth form for four or five years, attempting every year to win the single Barbados Scholarship. It was rare to have the Barbados Scholarship go to a science student, and it had never gone to a girl. I recall the shock when a girl from Queen's College won the coveted scholarship, which we all believed belonged almost by right to a Harrisonian. This tradition was reinforced visually, as there were boards in the assembly hall on which the names of the Barbados scholars were engraved in gold, and as schoolboys, we took pride in remembering the names of the giants going back to 1916, every one of us hoping that one day we would be numbered among the greats.

The Higher School Certificate Examination, on the basis of which the Barbados Scholarship was awarded, was normally taken in the upper sixth form, and boys indicated on entering for the examination whether they wished to compete for the Barbados Scholarship. The proxime to the Barbados Scholar received the Armstrong Memorial Scholarship prize of two hundred pounds. Three of us who were promoted from the fifth form to the lower sixth form progressed so well that we were allowed to take the Higher School Certificate Examination after one year. My mother encouraged me to enter the Barbados Scholarship as well, since it cost nothing. I declined, thinking that it would be arrogance on my part to compete with my elders and betters. When the results of the examination were returned, I was proxime to the Barbados Scholars, but because I had not entered for the scholarship, I could not receive the Armstrong Memorial Prize. My mother was furious, in part because we could well have done with the two hundred pounds. The next year, however, I did win a Barbados Scholarship and went to the university of my choice. Much was expected of me, and the letter of recommendation from my headmaster, J.C. Hammond, to the university registrar on 30 December 1950, which I still treasure, reads: "Alleyne is obviously a boy of outstanding ability, and his School record has been consistently brilliant. He is also of sound character and has been a reliable prefect."

CHAPTER 2

Growing up in Jamaica and Becoming West Indian
The University College of the West Indies

I elected to go to the University College of the West Indies at Mona, Jamaica, and study medicine. This caused some local consternation, as I was the first Barbados Scholar to opt to attend the fledgling university college. I say opt because Edson Inniss, who won a Barbados Scholarship the same year I did, was already at Mona on an exhibition. Why did I do it? I think my father would have been delighted had I elected to go to Britain, as most Barbados scholars had done. But several of my friends and colleagues were going to Jamaica or were there already. Some of them had entertained me with pictures of the social life there, and the local resident tutor, a Mr Douglas Smith, had painted an idyllic picture of the Valley of Mona and the richness of Jamaica life.

But I think the major reason was a nascent West Indian nationalism. I knew that the social structures of Tom Brown's schooldays or Wodehouse's Jeeves and Bertie Wooster were not for me, and to move from the white domination of Barbados to the white domination of Britain seemed not very smart. In addition, I heard Jamaica was a much more open society. Proximity was not an issue for us, as Jamaica was perhaps figuratively farther than Britain. I think my mother was secretly pleased, however, that I elected not to go to Britain, as I would not be tempted to marry a white girl and be subject, on return to Barbados, to the problems of a mixed marriage. I wonder if she ever thought of my marriage to a half-Chinese girl as a mixed one. If she did entertain such thoughts, she never voiced them. The college was established in 1948,[1] and it did not escape me that this was the hundredth anniversary of the Communist manifesto, much of which as a schoolboy I had read and internalized. Finally, I had heard and read of the possibility of a West Indian federation, and it struck me that a West Indian university could be central in the formation of a West Indian polity.

It was about time for me to leave home anyway. My father had difficulty seeing me as a young adult in his home; his concept of a home allowed for only one adult male. But at the end, his generosity of spirit is something I will always cherish – acknowledging my maturity by inviting me to have a rum and ginger with him at a party just before I left and telling me how proud he was of me and how much he loved me. I left from Seawell Airport on Friday, 5 October 1951, and that was the last time I saw him – erect, holding my mother's hand, as tears streamed down her face – watching their first child dressed in his brown tropical suit, US$200 pinned to his inside coat pocket, leave on the plane for Jamaica. It was for them all the more momentous, as neither of them had ever left Barbados.

THE MONA CAMPUS AND REFLECTIONS

My airplane travel to Jamaica on an ancient British West Indian Airways Dakota 3 was, of course, a novelty, and it was then that I met Archie Hudson-Phillips and Knox Hagley, who have remained among my best friends. My arrival in Jamaica was memorable – we were met by some undergraduates, driven to Mona, and, after being settled in Irvine Hall, we were taken to the junior common room, where I was firmly put in my place by one student. On being asked how long he had been there, he haughtily replied that he was a fourth-year medical student (with the accent on *medical*). I almost addressed him as "sir". But it was the physical environment of the campus that enthralled me. The fields around were covered in blinking fireflies, and on the radio, a popular singer, Jo Stafford, was singing "No Other Love", the music for which comes from Chopin's Etude No. 3 in E Major. Then I looked up to the hills, where I could see the blinking lights of the town of Newcastle. I could have sworn those were the lights of Jacob's ladder leading from this earth to heaven.

Indeed, one would have been dull of soul not to be entranced by the physical beauty of the Valley of Mona. There were wide green spaces, the enchanting fireflies, numerous mango and other trees; and the Blue Mountains were never just blue. They changed colour with the light and season, and no undergraduate could have been immune to the moon rising over those mountains. From the more densely populated part of campus, such as the halls of residence, one could see it rise and then hurry to the valley through which the old Hope River meandered and see it rise again. There was also the attraction of the Jamaican people themselves – their speech, their music, their dance. I stood mesmerized when I saw a group of men digging a ditch with their pickaxes rising and falling in unison, one man waving a small stick like a baton and running up and down the line, maintaining the rhythm and beat from a traditional digging song. I was fascinated by the imagery of the Jamaican expressions and would sometimes go to the Papine market on Friday afternoons just to listen to the richness of the banter and exchange between the market women as they used metaphors and similes and constructions that one would not find in a thesaurus but that conveyed precisely what they meant to say – which was not always complimentary.

The college began in an old army camp, which had previously served several purposes including being the temporary home for some of the European Jews escaping Hitler. Originally all students were housed in wooden huts, while the more substantial structures were being built, but a hurricane a couple months before I arrived had set back the construction considerably. We were lodged in Irvine Hall, which had four blocks of dormitories, two for male and two for female undergraduates.

I suppose it is inevitable that much of what is written about the early years of the university college turns around the personalities of both professors and students. It is common, for example, to find detailed reference to the striking personality and characteristics of Professor Norman Millott, the professor of zoology who did not write books. He was ambidextrous and would amaze students by his ability to draw detailed diagrams with his right hand and almost simultaneously label them with his left. There are many stories of his insistence on punctuality – the door to the lecture theatre being closed promptly as he began his lecture and late-comers having to sit on the steps outside and just listen. The story goes that on one occasion when he himself was a few minutes late, he found the door of the lecture theatre locked. I don't recall the consequences. There was Dr Francis Bowen, not noted particularly for his scholarship but beloved by all students for his generosity and his paternalistic interest in their welfare.

Dr Bowen would play an important role in my extracurricular life, as he persuaded me and several of my fellow undergraduates to become Freemasons. Becoming a Freemason was especially ironic for me, as in Barbados my father could not do so since the lodge he wished to join was reserved for whites only. I loved the beauty of the ritual, and I related to the principles of truth, fidelity, honour and generosity which were espoused as the essentials of a good life. I was enchanted by the camaraderie and the good fellowship that characterized our meetings. I also got to travel all over Jamaica with Dr Bowen to meetings of the various lodges and was fascinated by the warmth and hospitality with which we were greeted. I eventually became master of our university lodge, and even today I remember with affection those with whom I shared the Masonic experience.

The free and easy relationship between the staff and students struck me. The formality of lectures did not inhibit social interaction, and several staff members opened their homes to undergraduates for discussions that would range well beyond the academic. Perhaps it was because many of the staff themselves had graduated not that long ago.

I have often reflected on the impact of the institution itself on me as a young person and the clash between its environment and the environment from which I came. Apparent contradictions often played themselves out in my behaviours and anxieties in ways I did not fully understand at the time. Barbados in the early 1950s was a society still grappling with the possibility of the end of the colonial era. There was a strong religious ethic, with the church being the focal point for community activity and still being state supported. Racial divisions were an obvious part of everyday life and perhaps fell into that category of behaviour subsequently characterized, I am told, by Keith Hunte as apartheid practised by consenting adults. Moving from Barbadian society to a Jamaica in which whatever racial prejudice there was did not jar on the conscience, I felt relief or even escape. Jamaicans would say that there were divisions of class rather than colour, although one would hear of the hotels and beaches in Montego Bay, which did not admit blacks, but such divisions did not jar on the senses as they did in Barbados.

Discrimination in hotels existed not only in Montego Bay. We were told how as recently as 1948, a famous Jamaican journalist, Evon Blake, had created a major incident by desegregating the swimming pool of one of Jamaica's most prestigious hotels. The Myrtle Bank Hotel in Kingston was owned and operated by the United Fruit Company and was frequented almost exclusively by whites. Apparently on a hot summer day, Evon Blake stripped to his swimming trunks and jumped into the hotel pool. All of the white bathers immediately left, and there was chaos as this black man, smoking his pipe, swam around in the pool and dared them to evict him. We students were told that after he was persuaded to leave, the pool had to be drained and refilled, because it had been contaminated by a black person.

Jamaica also meant freedom from parental control. In Barbados, I had been under the control of my biological parents and indirect control of the many adults who acted *in loco parentis*. Adolescents have the urge to explore – they explore their bodies, their environment – and they often rub against the constraints imposed by the codes of behaviour that derive from the written and unwritten rules of the society. In Barbados, this exploration for me would have been inhibited by social and domestic constraints. To move from this restricted environment, marked by the strength of family bonds, to an environment so completely different, represented a shock.

While on the face of it there was considerable individual freedom, it became clear that institutional mores made patent the difference between freedom and licence. The formality that was present in the early days of the university was no doubt an expression of the institutional understanding of what was appropriate for young West Indians. The gowns students in the humanities wore to class and in interacting with the administration officials were part of that understanding. Similarly, the formality at dinners to which we wore gowns, the routine of afternoon tea, and the cleaning of the rooms by maids, all expressed the values of the university community.

The institution had the authority and imposed what was considered the behavioural orthodoxy of a good university college affiliated with a British university dedicated to producing a West Indian elite.

On the other hand, this new environment and its individual freedoms had to be considered in the context of academia as well as extramural life. To study well, one had to be self-disciplined, as indeed there were tremendous distracting pressures. The sophistication of much of the social life in Jamaica was something to which I had to adapt and adjust. Peer pressure came often from groups that were older; in the early years, many of the undergraduates were mature, having graduated from American or Canadian universities before entering the university college. There was pressure and freedom to explore tobacco and alcohol. Smoking was the norm, and alcohol consumption was an indication of masculinity. I had never smoked, and the sight of so many young women smoking was a revelation, as my mother regarded women who smoked to be of slightly loose morals. After a few weeks on campus, I found myself accepting cigarettes, then buying them to be able to offer them reciprocally. In addition, smoking was supposed to help one to study better. My association with tobacco came to an end when one night I fell asleep at my desk and awoke to find my zoology textbook open and a half-burned cigarette in the ashtray. My conclusion was that the habit was not for me – I really did not like it, it was expensive, it did not help me to study, and clearly it was a fire hazard. I never smoked again, and today when I am asked if I ever smoked, I answer yes, for three weeks, fifty-odd years ago.

The social distractions derived in part from freedom of access to various sites of entertainment – the students' union, the cinema – and especially the warm Jamaican hospitality. You only had to say that you were a university undergraduate, and you were immediately welcomed into homes. On one occasion Archie Hudson-Phillips and I spent two weeks' holiday with the Evans family. One day, we were being entertained by Mr Evans, a former minister of agriculture, and were fascinated by his discussion of the politics of the day, when suddenly he excused himself and went to his bedroom. It was the hour for the radio programme *Second Spring*, whose tag line was "Can a woman who has once loved completely ever find true love again?" Clearly, even politicians are not immune to radio love dramas.

Growing up in Jamaica and Becoming West Indian

The institutional orthodoxy and the contextual liberty produced tensions in newcomers to Jamaica, which sometimes played out in emotional and academic difficulties. There was a myth that every year at least one student had a severe mental health crisis. On one occasion I was impressed when the young professor of medicine Eric Cruickshank came to see a student who was uncontrollably manic. As the student approached menacingly, Professor Cruickshank expertly and almost professionally wrestled him to the ground and injected him with paraldehyde, which quieted him. Perhaps this is where I formed my impression that professors of medicine had to be men of valour and action.

Another of my enduring recollections of those early years is the degree of student involvement in the many activities and multiple societies. I recall almost constant opportunities for conversation. There were arguments about every considerable aspect of human endeavour, with politics and sport being preeminent. There was a palpable vibrancy to student life despite the small number of undergraduates who were truly polyvalent. There were or seemed to be innumerable clubs and activities, and numerous lectures on a wide variety of topics, and my recollection is of students from all faculties participating in them all. One memory is of arts students listening intently to a visiting urologist describe his special operation in which he shortened one of the pelvic muscles to restore male potency.

I was very involved in student politics and even contested the position of presidency of the Guild Council. I was defeated by Vincent Brown from Montserrat – he played the saxophone and was leader of the student band which played at most of the parties, even the formal ones. The band was not content with playing the standard tunes of the day and sometimes performed those composed by fellow students. One of these, "Mona Moon", has become a classic, redolent with remembrance of the magic of Mona. It is not well known that there were several other composers – men like Derek Walcott, who would become a world-renowned poet and win the Nobel Prize for Literature – who were inspired by their sweethearts to follow the time-honoured tradition of composing poetry to them. Owen Minott composed one such, and the first verse captures the spirit of that time.

> When it is moonlight
> I remember the perfume of your hair.
> When it is moonlight
> I can feel you so near.
> Why did you leave me, so lonely
> When you know how I care?
> Why did you leave me
> When I love you, my dear?

Actually, she never came back!

I did not have much time for reflection on the way there or in the early days in Jamaica. But from time to time now, I reflect on what got me there. First there was the sense of the importance of family in my development – a nuclear family with established roles. There was a security of there being a defined group to which one belonged and to which one owed allegiance and in some sense a responsibility. That closeness of family has persisted and perhaps grown stronger over the years, and I have developed an ever deeper appreciation of the value of the family as a unit of social organization. As a child, I had the advantage of not having competing attractions, so play, amusement and entertainment all revolved around the family. We did not exclude others, but those others were drawn into the family, strengthening rather than loosening the bonds.

My capacity to express myself and to articulate a coherent position did not come from my university education. It came from conversation around the table at meals. It came from my parents encouraging me at an early age to express myself and to argue my position. They allowed me to participate in adult debate, and one incident comes clearly to mind. There was a local debating society which was addressing the topic "The pen is mightier than the sword". The week before the debate, I pestered my mother with my views on the subject, so finally she said, "Why don't you get up and say so?" I recall standing on the chair that night in the school room and holding forth; for the life of me I cannot recall whether I argued for or against, but argue I did. The importance of family action also played itself out in the church. Both my parents were devout Christians – my mother was active in the church's social affairs, choir, and mothers' union. My father taught in Sunday School and was a lay preacher. Much of the religious dogma is not really vital to me now, but I believe that the relevance of many of the nostrums for a good society remain with me, and the centrality of the essential commandment *Do good and love ye one another* is one by which I try to live.

The discipline of primary and secondary school has also remained with me over the years. I have been asked if I had difficulty in medicine, having not done sciences in high school. My answer is that discipline is not theme specific. At a more prosaic level, I would contend that the precision and discipline of writing good Latin or Greek prose is easily transferable to medicine. Indeed, I still refer to some of the classics I learned in school. Aristotle's *Ethics*[2] and the thesis of proportionality continues to be useful as I speak, write and put into practice the notion of equity. Plato's concept of the thymotic part of the soul, which causes man to struggle, of which I read in Harrison College, is still relevant to my understanding of Francis Fukuyama's view of the inevitability of liberal democracy[3] in the search for global health equity.

The discipline of preparation, the essentiality of planning, the priority to be accorded to punctuality were all hard-wired into me during these critical years in school. As Martin Luther King Jr put it, human progress does not roll in on the wheels of inevitability.[4] I have referred to a love for reading. I often quote my father, whom I heard say that there were two things he wished he could bequeath to us that would always serve us well – "a love of books and a sense of humour". The latter is evident when we meet at family gatherings.

Now, as I look at some of my contemporaries, I am interested to note the success of those whose parents were schoolmasters like mine. There is Woodville Marshall, a distinguished historian, professor and pro-vice-chancellor of the University of the West Indies; Courtney Blackman, an economist and first governor of the Central Bank of Barbados; Oscar Jordan, a distinguished endocrinologist, founder of the Barbados Diabetes Foundation and of the Smith family – Vernon, Aurie, and Sir Frederick. We all were exposed to strict discipline, which was perhaps transposed from school to home. The emphasis was on scholarship and the ethos that it was not good enough just to be good enough: excellence was the expected norm.

THE FIRST YEAR OF MEDICINE

My first year was taken up with studying and passing chemistry, physics, zoology and botany. Since my knowledge of the subjects was rudimentary, it meant many long hours at my desk. I enjoyed the logic of physics, but perhaps because of the nature of the teaching, chemistry was something to be learned by rote. My artistic deficiencies weighed heavily on me in zoology; while some of my gifted contemporaries could spend a long time on their dissections because of their ability to draw rapidly and well, I had to hurry through my dissections and spend an inordinately long time drawing and labelling the specimens. I have to admit that my drawings often bore little resemblance to the careful dissections I had done. But I did manage to pass all the subjects and was promoted into the preclinical years.

During that summer of 1952 I paid my first visit to New York City. The process of obtaining a visa was a long and laborious one. There were photographs to be obtained, fingerprints to be taken, and notarized letters to be obtained from relatives in the United States demonstrating that they were financially capable of supporting me during the period of my stay. My friend Knox Hagley and I travelled from Kingston to Miami together. While waiting for the connection to New York, we went to an airport restaurant, where the white attendant took one quick look at us and said to the waitress, "Show them where to sit" – which was at the back of the restaurant. When I arrived in Brooklyn where my relatives lived, I was received suspiciously by my six male cousins, and though my natty dress of the red university blazer and cream flannel trousers did not impress them, we soon became fast friends. I was introduced to being addressed as "boy", having to wait to be served, helping an old person across the street and being offered a coin as a tip, and various other indignities which were the normal lot of black men and, I suppose, women. But I was also introduced to television for the first time and revelled in the jazz scene and life in general in New York. I saw live performances by many of the jazz greats of that era, such as Louis Armstrong, Dave Brubeck and Paul Desmond. Regardless of the activities on a Saturday night, Sunday morning church was mandatory. Much of the social life of my relatives, at least the older ones, revolved around the church, and I will never forget the fire-

and-brimstone preaching of gifted black ministers at eleven o'clock of a summer morning in a church without air conditioning. While in New York I became sensitive to the beginning civil rights struggle and was immersed in the literature of the Harlem Renaissance, which of course by then was over, but we still read and debated the work of Langston Hughes. There were books about freedom and justice everywhere, and arguments about them were often intense. The West Indian communities were vibrant, and one looked forward to the various picnics and boat rides sponsored by the sons and daughters of one or other island, on one of which I was mesmerized by the famous drummer Max Roach. I confess to a suspicion that there was more drive and striving for excellence among the offspring of West Indian immigrants than was seen in the blacks who had come from the South. When I would question them about certain behaviours which I thought unduly submissive, the answer would be that we could not understand, as although we might have had similar origins and a background of slavery, our recent experiences were vastly different. I suppose one only had to hear Billie Holiday sing "Strange Fruit" to appreciate the truth of their responses.

THE PRECLINICAL MEDICAL STUDENT

When I returned to Mona for my second year, I was placed in the new all-male Taylor Hall, comprising four blocks of forty single rooms each. There was intense rivalry between the halls, and even today, students of my era often identify themselves by their hall of residence. My medical student days were as uneventful or eventful as I suppose is the norm. There was the camaraderie of a small class, and five of us formed a close bond.

Knox Hagley was from Grenada: tall and handsome with a ready and engaging smile. He was a bit older than I was and had come from the prestigious Grenada Boys School, where he was influenced by a succession of Barbadian teachers. He had an excellent voice and was soon a member of the jazz band, where he became known for his rendition of "Mona Moon". He was a favourite of the ladies and made no secret that the admiration was mutual. Like most of us, he acquired a nickname. His was "Joseph", arising from his portrayal of Joseph in the annual nativity play. My contemporaries still recall turning his room into a small nightclub which we dubbed "Joe's Nitery" and which became famous for the exclusivity of its clientele. We prided ourselves that the Nitery hosted every batch of graduating nurses.

Cecil Bethel was from the Bahamas and came to the University College of the West Indies after having completed a degree at McGill University in Canada. He was the first Bahamian to attend the university college, and I suspect it was because his father had studied at Codrington College in Barbados and had several West Indian friends. He was the product of a social environment in Nassau which was more sophisticated than the one from which I came. He was always immaculately dressed, a keen sportsman, representing the university in tennis and basketball. I am not sure why he acquired the nickname of "Bony B", because bony he certainly was not.

Glen Nymn, from Tobago, was the quietest of us all. He had passed all the subjects required for the first year, so that year he did not have to take any examinations. I believe he had spent that time engaged in the many intense discussions about topics undergraduates discuss that have little relevance to academic work. He was the raconteur of the group and would regale us with improbable stories of life in Trinidad and Tobago. He measured everything, and once, having measured the inches of toothpaste in a tube, questioned the common room attendant about the number of tubes sold, as he had calculated how many inches would be used by the student body if everyone brushed regularly, using the same amount each time. He carried out a similar analysis for rolls of toilet paper. His nickname was "Fatso", because he was slim, muscular and an avid weightlifter.

James Ling was a Trinidadian, an island scholar from the prestigious Queen's Royal College, who had come to Mona after one year at McGill University in Canada. He was always dapper, and he introduced to us the Trinidadian penchant for pointed jokes – picong – and finding humour in the most peculiar situations. Because he was half Chinese, his nickname was "Mao", after Chairman Mao Tse Tung. His addiction was horse racing, and by all accounts he did well at it, even as a student and later a young doctor.

We five argued about everything under the sun, particularly politics, sport and women, partied vigorously, studied hard, graduated eventually and have remained fast friends.

Growing up in Jamaica and Becoming West Indian

There was perhaps some value to my classical background, as it got me into the good graces of my professor of physiology, Ian Mackay. I remember him as an affable, student-friendly teacher whose lectures were often tedious. One day in class, he was trying to explain an aspect of logical reasoning in relationship to some physiological principle. He put the question as to the meaning of the teleological approach (explaining the phenomenon by the purpose it serves) to one of the students, Bert Reese. Bert, rather mischievously, I think, replied that it was the art of being tedious. The question was passed to me, and in retrospect I must have appeared nerdish, but I gave the Greek origin of the word, which pleased the professor enormously. It would be rash to say that a lack of classical training contributed to Bert Reece failing physiology and dropping out of medicine.

My second and third years were different from the first. I had become more worldly wise, or perhaps Jamaica wise, and had spent a summer in New York City with relatives and returned understanding much more acutely the problems and practice of racial discrimination at a level I had not encountered even in Barbados. I had a serious conversation with myself at the end of the second year, however, by which time my academic interest had taken second place to the many blandishments offered within and outside of the university; I was an active participant in the many aspects of campus life. My wiser self got the better of the conversation, and I began to devote more time to my studies and eventually passed my second MB examination in the prescribed time. Our teaching then moved to the University College Hospital of the West Indies.

There were outstanding teachers. The professor of anatomy, Walter Harper, was a dour Scot whom I cannot remember ever seeing smile. He did not countenance frivolity in the dissecting room and impressed, at least on me, that the cadavers we dissected were human remains and should be treated with the appropriate respect. Much of anatomy was rote learning, and I discovered that the secret was to try to visualize the body in three dimensions and form a visual image of the relationships in that manner. I was helped in this by a remarkable local doctor, Dr Escoffrey, who also lectured in anatomy and who had the ability to draw in three dimensions on the blackboard. Of course, there were legends of students committing the whole of the anatomy textbook to memory, and of one who went to the examination and wrote so much on one question that he just managed to get through it and pass.

Physiology was much more logical, and I was fascinated with experiments on frogs – for example, eliciting and recording muscle response from nerve stimulation. In later years I got to appreciate that several of the explanations we learned of physiological functions were incorrect, but such is the nature of science with its constant unfolding of the secrets.

Pharmacology was absorbing not only because of the subject itself but because of the personality of our lecturer, Dr Paul Feng, who seemed to be interested solely in his work. The story goes that when he suffered a heart attack and was in intensive care, a resident came to give him some drug or other. He stopped the resident and quizzed him on the drug's mode of action and side effects, and reminded him of what he had been taught in pharmacology class a few years before.

THE CLINICAL YEARS

There was a tendency for the medical students in their clinical years to stick together, earning the reputation of being supercilious and condescending because of the white coat and stethoscope, which we wore both for functional purposes and as badges of status. The friendships of our small class of twenty-two were close then and remain so today. This does not mean that it was all study – we played poker and dominoes, and paired with Cecil Bethel, I won the only championship of my life to date – the annual university bridge tournament.

As is a tradition with medical students, there was an attraction for nurses. The University College Hospital of the West Indies was opened in 1953, in our second year, and because the nurses' hostel was incomplete, they were housed in Chancellor Hall. Those of us who lived in Taylor Hall could not help but be distracted by the stream of young, nubile females passing before our eyes every day as they walked to and from the hospital. When the nurses' hostel was completed, it was appropriately termed the Bastille. Campus lore is full of tales of intrepid males storming the Bastille.

I eventually fell in love with one of those nurses, Sylvan Chen, much to the delight of my mother and uncle and all my friends. The fact that she was Chinese never seemed to concern my family, although her Jamaican-Chinese relatives were initially lukewarm. My courtship did not begin well. As an arrogant fourth-year student in my first surgical rotation, I was called one day to the casualty or emergency room to suture a wound. I took up the syringe to draw the local anaesthetic, and a young nurse dutifully held up the bottle. Just as I was about to insert the needle into the cap, she pulled it back and said firmly, "You should read the label first." I was furious. Who was this young nurse to correct a fourth-year medical student? Of course, she was right. And that was my introduction to Sylvan.

I was curious about her, and one thing led to another and another. My mother was emphatic in reminding me that both our fathers had died, leaving families to be raised by the mother, and suggesting that this placed on me an obligation not to play carelessly with her affections. Eventually I found myself eyeing her and her alone, and I still remember clearly taking her back to the nurses' hall one night and, with tears in my eyes, asking her to marry me. I cried when she said yes. We became engaged on her twenty-first birthday, and I presented her with a ring that my sister Cynthia had bought for me in the duty-free shop in Curaçao. When I look at it now, I need a microscope to see the diamond, but it was what I could afford then, and today, when I can afford a real rock, she still will not change it.

When in early 1958 I discussed with her mother a possible date for our marriage, I suggested that we wait until the end of 1959, by which time I would have finished a post-internship year and be ready to go back to Barbados. Her mother said nicely that it would be best not to wait too long and that we should get married in December. I demurred, but, of course, it happened as her mother had "suggested", and we were married at the end of my internship, in December 1958.

As medical students, we were fortunate to have excellent clinical teachers. The emphasis was very much on clinical skills, using the senses to make a diagnosis. We learned that a patient's illness was the culmination of the impact of physical, environmental and social factors, and our professor of pathology emphasized the difference between disease and illness. He would say that disease is objective; it is the manifestation of abnormality in an organ or organs leading to functional change. Illness is a subjective phenomenon; it is the feeling engendered from having a disease. Of course, too much can be made of the distinction, as I learned subsequently. We were taught that the patient history and the detailed physical examination were the bases of the diagnosis and that the laboratory tests were ancillary or confirmatory. Eric Cruickshank, who was an avid bird-watcher and had an uncanny eye for detail, would teach that a physician should cultivate an ability for careful observation of external appearances such that one should have a fifty per cent chance of diagnosing the problem on first contact with the patient. There was banter between those who were interested in the art of medicine and those who preferred what was looked at then as the blood and guts of surgery. It is only much later that most of us would embrace the dictum of a famous surgeon – that an excellent surgeon is a good internist who knows when and how to cut. One of the exemplary teachers was the professor of surgery, Gerald Ovens, who was Mr Punctuality himself. He suffered multiple heart attacks and was so frustrated by his inability to operate that he became depressed and eventually committed suicide by dissecting out and cutting his femoral artery – the large artery that can be felt in the groin. Our class lore is that he so loved us that even after death, he sent us a message: the first question on our final surgery exam paper was related to the anatomy of that area.

There was excellent classroom teaching by first-rate professors and lecturers, and hands-on experiences, and I can still recall the joy at helping to deliver a baby, the pleasure at seeing a patient recover from pneumonia with penicillin, the new miracle antibiotic, at standing on the other side of the operating table and feeling that I was part of a healing process, at making a correct diagnosis and being complimented for having done so. But I reserve a special place in my memory for the extramural teaching and practice, which stands out in part because much of it is associated with John Golding, the orthopaedic surgeon who was senior lecturer and later became professor of orthopaedics. A model of patient-centred care, he lectured to us on ethics and practised what he taught. He would take us to visit other hospitals with him and involve us in the management of patients outside the university's hospital.

THE POLIOMYELITIS EPIDEMIC OF 1954

During a morning lecture on orthopaedics in 1955, in one of the old wooden classrooms in the hospital, John Golding announced to our small class that he needed our help. The poliomyelitis epidemic that began in 1954 was overwhelming the capacity of the health system.[5] The records show that during the course of the epidemic, there were 759 paralytic cases with 94 deaths, and John had worked heroically to establish a rehabilitation centre in the Mona Valley, to which he sent the recovering cases. This was later to become a major rehabilitation centre and a focal point for Physical Medicine in the Caribbean, and it still bears his name. But at the height of the epidemic, his urgent need was for physiotherapists, as there were just not enough of them to treat the flood of patients and to put them through the various exercises critical for their recovery. Many of my classmates and I volunteered, taking a crash course in elementary physiotherapy before we could treat the patients.

I will always remember the difficulty I had in maintaining my composure and a cheerful face in dealing with some patients and their problems. There was one in particular who tore at my deepest emotions. He was a popular, handsome, articulate, gifted athlete, who felt with justification that he had the chance to emulate the great Jamaican middle-distance runners like Arthur Wint and Herbert McKinley. After the acute phase of the disease was over, he had to come to terms with the reality of the paralysis of his lower limbs and the fact that he would never don spikes again. As I exercised him, he would rail against fate and wonder why he and not others less gifted had been struck down. Neither sympathy nor empathy would quench the fires of his anger or his tendency to lash out verbally at even those whom he must have known were being helpful. That was my first real lesson in dealing with an angry patient, and I was not yet experienced enough, nor did I have the communication skills needed to encourage the patient's compliance. It was difficult not to personalize the anger, to realize that he had to process and deal with his frustration, which he probably did not understand. The necessary communication skills and the facility for compassion and empathetic listening would come to me much later.

THE GROOMING OF A CHANCELLOR

THE KENDAL TRAIN CRASH

It was very late on the Sunday evening of 1 September 1957. I had taken Sylvan to the movies and on return was studying in my room, as final examinations were to begin in October. Sometime after midnight, I heard a knock on my door and opened it to John Golding. I was shocked, of course, as one's professors do not normally come calling at those hours. In typical fashion he apologized for disturbing me and said that there had been a horrible train wreck in Manchester. He was going there and was taking his registrar, Ronald Berry, and his assistant who made the plaster casts, Mr Brown. Would I like to come with them? Who could resist such an invitation? We set off to Kingston in his car to join a train which would take us to the site of the crash at Kendal. It was always an experience to drive with John, as like Jehu, the son of Nimshi, "He driveth furiously."

A train filled with Catholic churchgoers from Kingston had been to Montego Bay on an excursion, and on its way back was horribly overcrowded. In subsequent accounts, it was claimed that hordes of criminals and pickpockets joined the devout church people, and so riotous and raucous was the behaviour that a priest predicted God would wreak vengeance on the ungodly among them. No one can vouch for the immediacy of divine intervention, but the train derailed at Kendal in Manchester, killing two hundred persons and leaving seven hundred injured. It was the worst disaster in Jamaican history and the second worst rail crash in the world to that date.[6]

On reaching the scene, I saw what I imagined a battlefield would be like. There were corpses strewn all over the ground; there was weeping and wailing from the onlookers. Parenthetically, I was interviewed by a reporter at the crash site, my only appearance on the BBC. Sylvan's mother heard it and called her excitedly, but also with a bit of incredulity, to say I was being interviewed at the site of a world-shaking event.

John soon decided that we would be most useful in treating the injured, so off we went to the nearby Spalding's hospital, where John joined Dr Rob, the local surgeon. John taught me to take and develop x-rays, and when it was decided that it was time to operate on those who needed it, and these were mainly amputations, I assisted him in one theatre as the anaesthetist, while other members of his team were similarly engaged in other theatres. Here was I, a final-year medical student just a month away from my exams, anesthetizing patients at one end of the operating table while my professor was taking off legs at the other. What has remained with me is the need, in such a crisis, to process data quickly and take decisions. I was impressed by the speed and certainty with which John acted and ever grateful for his confidence in my ability to stand up to the obvious pressure that the occasion engendered.

Here is John's description of the event:[7]

> None of us, for instance is likely to forget Dr Vincent Rob in Spaldings. I will think of him as I saw him on the day of the Kendal rail disaster which left over a hundred dead on the track, and the hospitals at Mandeville and Spaldings overflowing with the injured. I had received a telephone call at 4 am to assemble a team to go immediately to the railway station in Kingston where a train was waiting to take us to Mandeville. Sam Street was getting another team together from KPH [Kingston Public Hospital].
>
> I got my Registrar, plaster man and our students ready – one of whom was (now Sir) George (Champ) Alleyne –and set off in my car at breakneck speed. We got to the site of the disaster just after dawn. It was an unreal site which met our eyes: a lovely cool morning, the bees gently buzzing around and with dead bodies draped over the overturned carriages as though they were supposed to be there. The injured had already been taken to Mandeville or Spaldings. Sam went to Mandeville and I took my group off to Spaldings.

An episode of hospitalization (which does not appear in my curriculum vitae) was memorable as being the only occasion on which I was undisciplined enough to take my own discharge against medical advice. I developed an infection between my toes, which led to a high fever, a painful swollen leg and swollen, tender inguinal lymph nodes from an ascending lymphangitis. My friend Knox took me to the emergency room of the hospital, where I was examined by the doctor and a series of officious clinical medical students, one of whom declared knowledgeably that I was probably suffering from some venereal disease. I was admitted to the hospital ward and examined by Dr Ken Stuart, then a registrar, who eventually became Professor Ken Stuart, and he prescribed intramuscular penicillin every six hours. This was before the advent of disposable needles, and our used needles were sharpened and reused. I still believe that a couple of my injections were given by a nurse who did not care for me for various reasons unrelated to medicine, and all the needles she used seemed to have hooks at the end. They hurt going in, and they hurt coming out. After about the third injection, I called for my clothes and, to the consternation of the ward sister, signed my discharge and decided that if there was a choice between penicillin injections and the risk of death from septicaemia, I would take the risk. I did take it and I survived.

Of the many dramatic events of these years, that of a female lecturer who attempted suicide stands out. Apparently because of unrequited love, she took an overdose of barbiturates and was admitted to hospital in a coma. John Waterlow, then a lecturer in physiology, heard of the case and recalled reading in the journal *Nature* of a chemical – beta beta methylethyl glutarimide – which had been shown to reverse the narcotic effect of barbiturates.[8] Of course, this was not a drug available in Jamaica. He called the professor of chemistry, Cedric Hassell, and asked if he could synthesize the chemical locally. Hassell agreed, and he and his students went to the laboratory, worked through the night and synthesized the chemical. It was given to the patient, and she recovered miraculously. History does not recall what happened to her love life thereafter.

In our final years, we did work hard, and we graduated with degrees from the University of London, with which our University College of the West Indies was in special affiliation at that time. The student magazine, the *Pelican*, in describing our class, had this to say of me: "A Barbados scholar, he is one of the brighter students in his class. Has many interests, chiefly sports – cricket, tennis, football. Has served on the Guild Council. A vivacious conversationalist. Succeeds in mixing work and play."

I think that was a pretty fair assessment. I won the Allenbury Prize in Clinical Medicine, won the silver medal as the best student in clinical medicine and graduated top of my class with the gold medal as the best student.

Growing up in Jamaica and Becoming West Indian

BECOMING A WEST INDIAN IN THE UNIVERSITY

My undergraduate years were happy ones. I matured emotionally, learned how to organize the various parts of my social and academic life, and appreciated how to live in the community of persons from different backgrounds. I learned the need for financial responsibility and after my father's death would help my mother with such savings as I could muster from my scholarship. But perhaps most importantly, I became a West Indian. I know from the record that the idea behind the establishment of the university was to create locally a cadre of West Indian leaders, as the West Indian leaders who existed had mostly been formed in metropolitan centres. History has shown that this original purpose has been fulfilled. Many of my friends and perhaps the majority of students at Mona of that era have said that they acquired a West Indian consciousness in those early days, and I have often wondered not at the veracity of the assertion but at its genesis. Why do I, we, speak of being proud to be West Indian? I often reflect on the processes and institutions that contributed to our being socialized into being West Indian.

The feeling of wishing to be a part of a new West Indian experience had motivated my going to Mona, but there was perhaps at that time a poorly formed and virtual notion of being West Indian. There must have been a socialization, which certainly did not come from our teachers, the vast majority of whom were expatriates, and I do not recall the few West Indians among them, at least in medicine, making West Indianism a reference point for their discourse. Any West Indian focus from elders would have come from visitors such as Eric Williams and from our reading about West Indian leaders. There were Sunday lectures by scholars like C.L.R. James, who dealt with subjects as diverse as Marx and Euripides. I heard him say once that if one wished to understand social changes in the West Indies, "You have to read Marx, you have to read Fanon and you have to read me."

In retrospect, the major agents of the socialization into being West Indian were peers, the media and perhaps sports. Peer culture is a critical factor in formation of identity. Our peers obviously did not set out to socialize us into being West Indian, as for the most part they were themselves being baked in the same oven. It was the discussion, the debate, the recognition of degrees of similarity and some differences, and the multiple physical and social interactions that contributed to the mutual establishment of the culture. And I am sure the arguments about the different viewpoints, but also the humour, sometimes pointed and bordering on the crude, contributed. Some of us wondered if this process was not more marked among the students from the South, but close examination shows that that was definitely not so. Some of the most fervent proponents of the West Indian ideal are Jamaicans of my era – men such as P.J. Patterson, Rex Nettleford, Lloyd Stanford, and women such as Gloria Samms-Knight. The media would have played a role, and I refer to not only the popular media but the entertainment media as well. I recall a concert on campus on the occasion of the celebration of the Jamaican tercentenary and one of the calypsonians singing: "The Tercentenary will always remain a page in Jamaica history / Jamaica, go marching on and on, one day you will reach Federation."

We were witnesses to the debates and discussions among the West Indian leaders about the shape of the federation, to which I was emotionally attached. I once earned the opprobrium of fellow Barbadians when in a radio interview I argued against situating the federal capital in Barbados, as I felt it would be stifled there by racism. I was not alone in this. The media were full of the debates about federation and the pros and cons of one or other form of organization. Most of my colleagues were interested in West Indian politics, and we followed, sometimes with concern, what seemed to us the ebb and flow of enthusiasm for the federation.

I was elated and almost euphoric at the conclusion of the 1956 London conference, at which the decision was taken that the West Indies would move forward in a federation, and definitive steps were taken to put the federal architecture in place. Sports contributed to that socialization, as we followed keenly the performance of the West Indies cricket team, and in spite of the vigorous criticism of selectors for one or other choice and debates on the relative merits of the players, there was unity of support for and identity with the team. There was a vibrant student press – the *Pelican* magazine and the *Pelican Annual* being the most professional. And there were also the cartoons, and the occasional "rags", such as *The Book of the Dead*, in which a particularly gifted and older student, Dunstan Champagnie, lampooned people and events in quasi-biblical prose.

It is interesting that the dissolution of the West Indies Federation did not lead to a desocialization and a renouncing of the notion of West Indianism in colleagues of my era. Those who were socialized into being West Indian at Mona in my day have remained committed to the ideal, which must of necessity find expression in ways other than through a political structure. The West Indies Federation foundered on the shoals of jealousy and insularity, and the short-sightedness of leaders who could not see beyond national parochial interests. I have contended that had the federation come into being when our political leaders were products of the university, then this spirit of West Indianism might have been a bond strong enough to overcome the fissiparous tendencies that played themselves out in the dissolution of the federal enterprise. It is one thing to have known a few colleagues in London or New York, but it is another to have spent several years in close contact with colleagues from other West Indian territories – played with them, laughed with them, drunk beer or rum with them, married some of them and formed bonds of the spirit with them.

CHAPTER 3

The Postgraduate Years
Internship

After graduation I spent the first six months of my internship in Professor Cruickshank's team and the second with a brilliant surgeon from British Guiana, Mr Harry Annamunthodo. It was initially a shock to appreciate that I was now a doctor with responsibilities for patients and that the decisions I made could affect their lives. It was difficult not to become emotionally engaged with patients and their relatives, noting their different reactions to illness. I saw a priest watch his young son die from leukaemia and was moved by the stoicism with which he comforted his wife and accepted it as God's will. One could never tell who would rail at the prospect of the nothingness of death and who would be comforted by the prospect of life after death and being reunited with their deceased loved ones. I remember Roger Mais, the celebrated Jamaican novelist, dying from cancer at age fifty, cursing God loudly in the most vivid language and almost demanding an explanation of why he who had so much to do was being allowed to die.

The therapeutic armamentarium was limited, and the only drugs which actually cured illness were the antibiotics. This was the dawning of the era of faith in man's ability to overcome infectious diseases forever. The absence of most of the sophisticated diagnostic tools made for acumen in clinical diagnosis. But in addition, because of the paucity of therapeutic tools, perhaps more attention was paid to giving care to patients throughout illness. Perhaps death was not regarded so much as defeat for the phy-

The Postgraduate Years: Internship

sician who appreciated that on occasion all he or she had to offer was care in its various aspects. There was care that involved making patients comfortable physically, and there was care through empathy during the times of stress and uncertainty which are the normal accompaniments of illness. I learned that no one has the right to remove hope from a patient, and sometimes what might seem as pandering to whims was satisfying some of that hope. Many of these lessons were amplified during the succeeding years of clinical practice, but I remain ever grateful to physicians like Professor Cruickshank, who exemplified many of the characteristics I have mentioned.

Surgical internship under Mr Annamunthodo was fascinating, as the experience was completely different from that of being a student. There was an incredible feeling of awe, pride and some humility at being taught to remove an appendix or repair a hernia. It was quite obvious that cure in the sense of restoration to health was much more common in the surgical than in the medical wards. Mr Annamunthodo was the kindest of men and possessed an amazing dexterity compared to some of his less gifted surgical colleagues, who would take twice as long as he did for a procedure.

By now I was firmly convinced that my specialty would be internal medicine. I was attracted to medicine, because at that time it seemed more intellectually satisfying. I admired the thought processes that went into making a diagnosis. In addition, I believed that in internal medicine, more clearly than in other areas, one saw the disturbances of physiology leading to illness. So much for the arrogance of youth, because as I appreciated later, all disciplines exercise the same critical thinking. I was also influenced by the charisma of the then professor of medicine, Eric Cruickshank.

At the end of my internship, I spent an additional year in the pathology department as a junior pathologist, rotating through various departments such as haematology and chemical pathology. We were on call for examining specimens taken during the night, and this sometimes led to unusual requests. One of our lecturers was interested in some aspect of the pancreas of diabetic patients who died. As the junior pathologist, I was on a couple occasions summoned to remove the pancreases of patients who had died at night. Entering a morgue alone in the dead of night to perform a limited autopsy called for steady nerves and lack of a belief in ghosts.

I planned to return to Barbados in January 1960, but that had to be postponed, as it turned out, by circumstances in which I almost caused my wife's death.

On the morning we were due to depart, she complained of feeling unwell, and my response was that she was nervous because she was going to meet new relatives and leaving the comfort of her home, and I advised her to pull herself together. However, our neighbour, a classmate of mine, on coming to say goodbye, noticed that she was a bit pale and that her abdomen was distended. In fact, she had a ruptured ovarian cyst, her abdomen was filled with blood, and she had to have emergency surgery. Had she taken my advice and boarded the plane to Barbados, she certainly would have died before we reached there. Since then, I have been reluctant to give advice to her or other members of my family about matters medical.

THE BARBADOS GENERAL HOSPITAL

Eventually we did travel to Barbados, where I worked in the Barbados General Hospital as a medical officer under a superb physician, Harold Forde. In my first week at work, I reported to the chief medical officer, Dr Maurice Byer, who gave me a lesson which I have never forgotten. He enquired what I wished to do and learned that I intended to spend a year or two in Barbados, apply for government support and proceed to Britain to do my postgraduate examinations in internal medicine. He listened carefully and then advised me as follows: "Dr Alleyne, I wish you to remember always that institutions are very impersonal things, but like living organisms their main function is to survive. Remember that they have nothing against you, but also they have nothing for you. So never rail against the government because its actions do not fit with your personal desires."

There were no interns in the hospital at that time, only we six junior doctors, who also took our turns as casualty officers at night and on weekends. There were two registrars and several consultants, most of whom were engaged primarily in their private practices. On many nights, I was the only doctor in the hospital. This was not ideal, but I acquired a wealth of experience, which has stood me in good stead. My patients included adult males and females with a wide range of infectious and non-infectious disease, children, the majority of whom were malnourished, and even the occasional psychiatric problem. I even spent a few months as the acting resident government pathologist, which caused Sylvan much worry, as I undertook forensic work of which I had only the most elementary knowledge. I recall with gratitude the incredible experience of the nurses and appreciated that if I was appropriately humble and willing to learn, I could benefit enormously from their accumulated practical wisdom and experience. The sister of one of my wards, Sister Crane, was an amazing diagnostician, and when it came to venepuncture, I swear she could draw blood from a stone.

These years taught me much. First, there was the lesson of self-reliance. Because of the nature of the institution, which was grossly understaffed by modern standards, I had to take many decisions which normally would have been made at higher levels in the professional hierarchy. I learned to trust my judgement but also learned when I had to ask for advice. I also improved my capacity to manage conflict, even although in many cases I did not appreciate I was doing so. I learned to accommodate or perhaps pander to the whims of prima donna physicians in order to get the best done for my patients. There was tension between the heads of various specialties, and it required considerable diplomacy to get the best advice for my patients even when the consultant giving the advice did not appreciate from whom the request came.

Some of my most poignant medical experiences occurred during this period, and one I recall vividly is that of holding in my arms a young man with sickle-cell anaemia, who in addition had developed severe acute rheumatic fever and cardiac failure. He held on to me tightly with tears in his eyes and implored me not to let him die.

I do not believe I have ever worked as hard as I did during the time I spent at the Barbados General Hospital. I would be on shift sometimes for thirty-six hours, come home, and after supper spend several hours reading medical journals and the postgraduate textbooks I knew I would need. Sometimes I drank coffee to stay awake and then took thalidomide to sleep.

I was intent on proceeding to London to take my Membership of the Royal Colleges of Physicians (MRCP) examination, which at that time was an essential prerequisite to being a specialist in internal medicine. The older heads and sundry government officials tried to persuade me to wait a few years, but Sylvan was even more insistent than I that we should go to London as soon as possible. On one occasion when the suggestion to wait was made in her presence, she retorted that we were going even if we had to tie two shoes together and row across the Atlantic Ocean. Sylvan had recovered completely and worked as a research assistant for Kenneth Standard, who was investigating the nutritional status of schoolchildren. She also worked part-time as a nurse in Nestlé's mothercraft service, counselling new mothers on infant nutrition. My time in Barbados was also marked by my mother's first stroke. Eventually she made an amazing recovery after being unconscious for about one week. During her illness, Sylvan was mother to my three youngest sisters – a period which they still recall with fondness.

LONDON

Eventually I obtained a Glaxo Fellowship of one thousand pounds, and with the little money we had saved, particularly from Sylvan's work as a mothercraft nurse, we left for Britain. The letter of approval of my leave gave me two years and $576 from the Training Scheme Fund. My plaintive letter of August 1961 asking for further financial assistance evoked no response. On Professor Cruickshank's recommendation, I had been accepted on the medical unit of University College London as a supernumerary registrar to Professor Max Rosenheim, whom I had met in Jamaica when he was the external examiner in medicine for our final examinations. I was fortunate that Prem Ratan, who was two years my senior, had occupied a similar position and had left a favourable impression.

We left Barbados in September 1961 on the SS *Golfito*, made a brief stop in Jamaica, and eventually reached Southampton after a rough passage in which a Scottish engineer tried to persuade Sylvan that brandy was the ideal remedy for seasickness. We were met by the British Council and taken to a hotel in Earl's Court until we could find accommodation. We still joke about the grey of the "white" bedsheets and the proximity of the floor as we lay in bed. We also discovered that scrambled eggs swam in a milky liquid and that rhubarb pie was an acquired taste.

The Postgraduate Years: Internship

Eventually, after being rejected by various landlords and landladies because of my colour, we met a most gracious Jewish couple, the Melkmans, who let us a floor of their home. We have fond memories of their home at 24 Hillfield Road in Hampstead, including inviting our Professor Rosenheim to dinner one evening, much to the amazement of my colleagues at our presumptuousness. Sylvan had prepared a splendid dinner, which was almost ruined by my nearly dropping the roast chicken on the floor and bringing out overripe Camembert cheese after dinner. The Melkmans were strict orthodox Jews who had escaped from Poland before the holocaust and were exquisitely sensitive to matters of racism or discrimination. After we left, they took in several other West Indian couples whom we recommended.

Before arriving in London, my intention had been to sit for my MRCP examination sometime in 1962 or 1963 after following the tried pattern of taking various preparatory courses. But my friend Kenneth Standard, who came to Britain soon after we did, challenged me to take the exam three months after arriving and offered to pay half the entrance fee if I did. This was hubris in the extreme, but Professor Rosenheim encouraged me and arranged for me to take an evening course at the Whittington Hospital. I also studied hard and counted on the extensive clinical experience I had acquired in Barbados under Harold Forde. Suffice it to say, I took up Kenneth's offer and passed the examination at my first attempt, which was unusual, since of the nearly three hundred people who entered the first of the four stages of the examination, only eleven of us survived. Only two of us passed on the first attempt. I still recall one of the eleven who passed being chagrined, if not annoyed, that this foreign black fellow had passed on the first attempt, when he, an Englishman, had needed seven attempts to do so.

My final oral examination at the Royal College of Physicians was an impressive affair. I sat at the foot of a long, baize-covered table around which the censors sat, with the whole proceedings being presided over solemnly by the president of the college. I usually did well in oral examinations, because I took the view that once the examiner had posed the question, he was in a sense at my mercy, and it is difficult for an examiner to stop a student who is fluent and making sense. It was also fairly easy to lead the examiner along a particular line of questioning in which I knew the answers. Suffice it to say that at the end of the oral, I was asked to wait in the secretary's office. After a brief interval, the college registrar came out and passed a slip of paper to the secretary. She looked up at me and said, "Congratulations, Dr Alleyne, you have passed." I was so overjoyed that I hugged and kissed her.

There was considerable myth and mystique around this examination. Legend had it that the candidate had to wear a grey three-piece suit, so I duly bought one. A particular story went that one candidate who had the temerity to wear a brown suit to his final oral examination was upset when on leaving, one examiner said to him, "Do enjoy your golf." He failed. Another story had it that an examiner smiled and said to the candidate at the end of the oral examination, "Please enjoy your day, as it is indeed a beautiful spring day. And just think that next spring you and I will be here to enjoy this kind of day again." I don't believe any of these apocryphal, rather sadistic tales.

After passing my MRCP, I continued to work in London, and these were glorious days for Sylvan and myself. I recollect sitting "in the gods" in the theatre in Golders Green, watching the Gilbert and Sullivan opera *HMS Pinafore*, seeing the opera *Aida* in Covent Garden, and discovering that Indian restaurants gave the best value for money. We saw snow for the first time, and I was deeply embarrassed when Sylvan's general practitioner diagnosed her chilblains and enquired what her husband did for a living. I experienced the change of affect that came with spring and could appreciate the words of Catullus:[1]

> Now spring brings back unchilled warmth
> Now the rage of the equinoctal sky
> Grows silent with the pleasant breezes of the west wind.

For most of the time on Professor Rosenheim's medical unit, I attended his ward rounds, helped to care for his patients and assisted in his out-patient clinics. He was a recognized authority on hypertension and renal disease, and here I began my interest in nephrology. I was fairly quickly accepted by my medical colleagues, though it was a bit more difficult to gain the confidence of the stern ward sister. But eventually I did, and she even invited Sylvan and me to dinner in her flat. Among various initiatives, I began a research project in the Medical Unit in University College on the electrolyte composition of the muscle of rats injected with steroids, but this produced no useful results, primarily because I knew little or nothing about research.

I was asked to be a locum registrar in the Hospital for Tropical Diseases, because it was assumed that coming from the tropics, I would have some expertise in this area. But the majority of the cases I saw there were completely different from those to which I had been accustomed in the Caribbean. They were mainly patients coming from Africa or Asia with the health problems peculiar to those areas. This served to confirm in my mind that the notion of tropical disease is irrelevant and disease patterns very much area specific. The experience was useful, however, as I did learn about new problems and unusual presentations of old ones. My residence in the hospital also confirmed my intense and persistent dislike for rhubarb pie, which seemed to be served for dessert every night.

I served as registrar for a short period in the Gerontology Unit under distinguished physician Lord Amulree, whose main strengths were his awareness of the social needs of his patients and his ability to connect with them on a deeply personal level. I came to appreciate keenly the nature of the social problems which contributed to much of the illness among the elderly in Britain. I could never have imagined that in an affluent society, one would come across elderly patients who existed on little else besides bread and tea for long periods of time. It also became clear to me that much of the disability of the elderly resulted from society failing to provide the support necessary for them to function adequately and independently.

One of the highlights of our stay in Britain was a visit to Cardiff at the invitation of Archie Cochrane, a distinguished epidemiologist who had virtually invented the randomized control trial as the gold standard for determining the effectiveness of interventions. He was instrumental in forming the Medical Research Council Epidemiology Unit in the university, and while I was an intern, I had attended to him when he became ill on a visit to Jamaica. He had been grateful for my care and insisted that we contact him when we came to Britain. He was an avowed communist, had fought against General Franco in the Spanish Civil War, and quite seriously suggested that I write to the Government of China, explaining that we had just escaped the British colonial yoke and wished to visit a progressive society. He assured me that we would be received and treated royally, but we had decided that this was an offer we should refuse.

We travelled by train to Cardiff, where we were received warmly by Archie and taken to his home. I found out that he was a rich bachelor, and his home was literally a castle, whose walls were hung with magnificent paintings and whose spacious gardens were filled with sculptures from some of Britain's most famous artists. He retained a large staff, and Sylvan and I dined on a silver service for the first and only time in our lives. We toured the Rhondda Valley, which was the field laboratory for much of his famous epidemiological research. One evening he took us for dinner to his favourite restaurant on the docks of Cardiff, where we ate well, drank far too much Pouilly-Fuissé and watched the waitresses and Archie dance on the table after dinner.

Among his famous publications is *Effectiveness and Efficiency: Random Reflections on the Health Service*,[2] an autographed copy of which he gave to me. He made it clear that he regretted I was training to be a physician. His terse comment was that perhaps I should do something useful with my life, such as study epidemiology and work in public health. His name is perpetuated in the now famous Cochrane Library, a collection of databases organized principally by the Cochrane Collaboration. The critical component is the collection of Cochrane reviews, a database of systematic reviews and meta-analyses which has become the cornerstone of evidence-based medicine.

While in London, we took the opportunity to visit my sister Cynthia and her husband Ronald in Marrakesh in Morocco. Ronald had qualified as a surgeon in Paris, had worked in Rabat and was a locum surgeon in Marrakesh. We exchanged telegrams about travel dates, and when they were fixed, we set off from London via Paris and Casablanca by air, and then to Marrakesh by train. Unfortunately, Ronald had forgotten to give me the address of their apartment and had just said that he would meet us at the train station. We arrived in Marrakesh about midday, but there was no Ronald. I spoke little French and no Arabic but said in jest to Sylvan that my father always told us that you would never be lost if you spoke English.

The Postgraduate Years: Internship

We took a horse drawn carriage, a *calèche*, to the police station and asked if they knew Dr Wilson. The confident response was that they did not know him, but if we returned at three o'clock, they certainly would have contacted him for us. As a backup, however, we decided we would make inquiries at the British Embassy. There we were graciously received, and the staff did trace Dr Wilson, who dutifully came and collected us. Just out of interest, a few days later we thought we would check at the police station and perhaps thank them. Interestingly, we received the same answer as before: "We don't know Dr Wilson, but if you come back at three o'clock, we certainly will have contacted him for you."

Exposure to the Arab culture and way of living was a marvellous experience. We explored the souk, visited the Atlas Mountains and were exposed to the technique of bargaining a fair price for something we wished. Purchase of a brass platter took several days, several cups of tea with the vendor and a number of visits to him with my sister, before the final price was settled. I was led to believe that it bordered on the vulgar to ask a price, accept it and pay without bargaining.

RETURN TO JAMAICA

I returned to Jamaica in October 1962 as senior registrar to Professor Cruickshank. There were four medical wards, two male and two female, and four teams, or firms. Each firm was headed by a consultant physician, and the rest of the team was a registrar, an intern and medical students. The registrar's duties consisted of organizing the work of the team, examining patients after they had been examined by the intern, and presenting them to the consultant, who confirmed or modified the diagnosis and line of treatment prescribed. Being registrar to the professor of medicine was reckoned to carry some status, and at that time, I was the only one with my MRCP, and I had more experience than the others. One of the other firms was headed by Professor Ken Stuart, a brilliant Barbadian physician who had carved out an impressive international reputation for his research in clinical medicine.

The year was uneventful clinically but very full socially. At the end of our time there, we visited my relatives in New York City and had a marvellous time. My aunts loved Sylvan, who was seeing the United States for the first time and who still recalls having her first taste of pizza. We did all the things tourists do, such as visiting the Empire State Building and the museums and taking a boat ride on the Hudson River. One of the highlights was a visit to the New York World's Fair and marvelling at the twelve-storey, stainless steel model of the earth called the Unisphere. We were intrigued by the domestic robots and the demonstration of kitchen equipment such as a ceramic cooktop stove. Many of these futuristic appliances are now in common use.

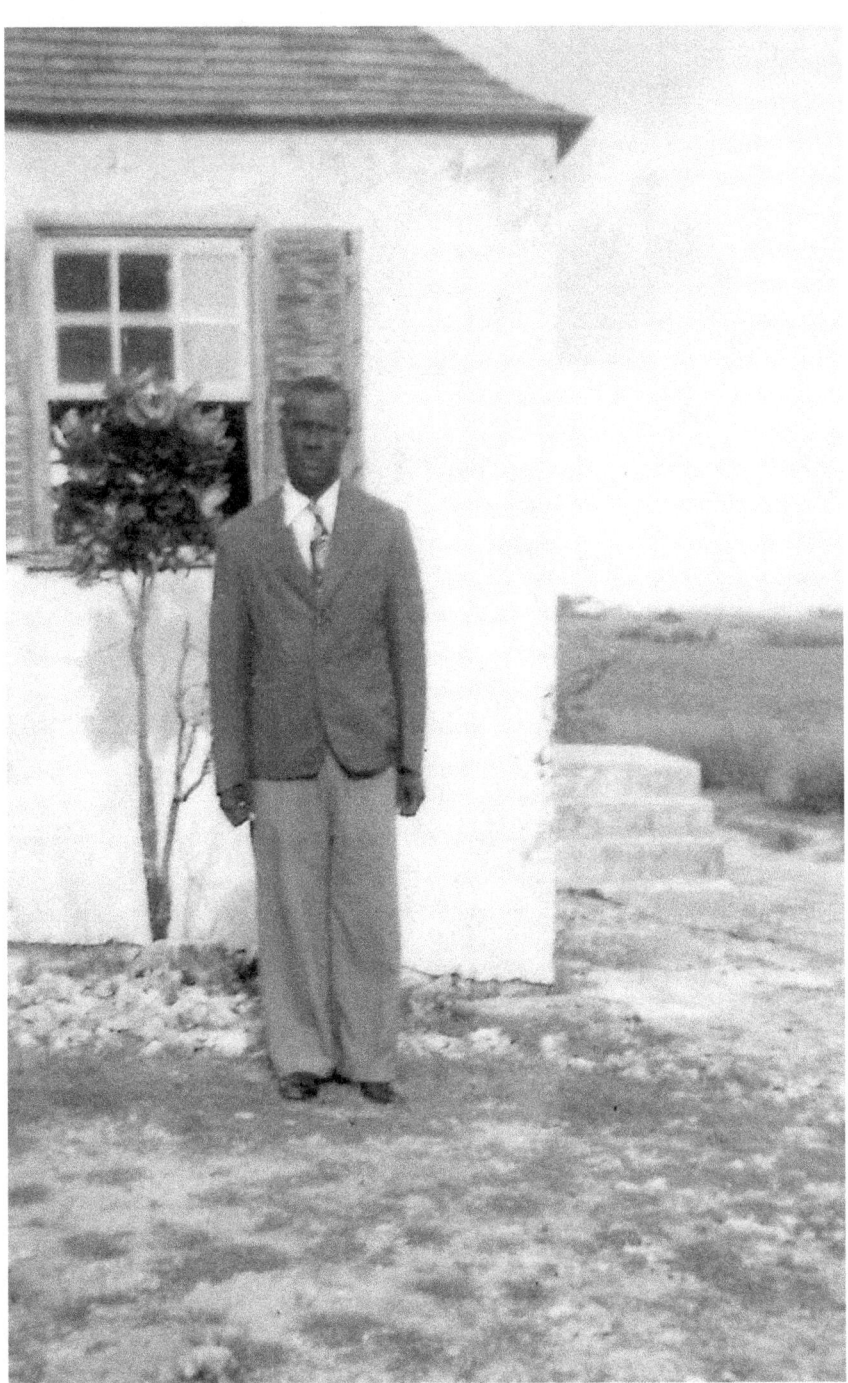

My father, Clinton Alleyne

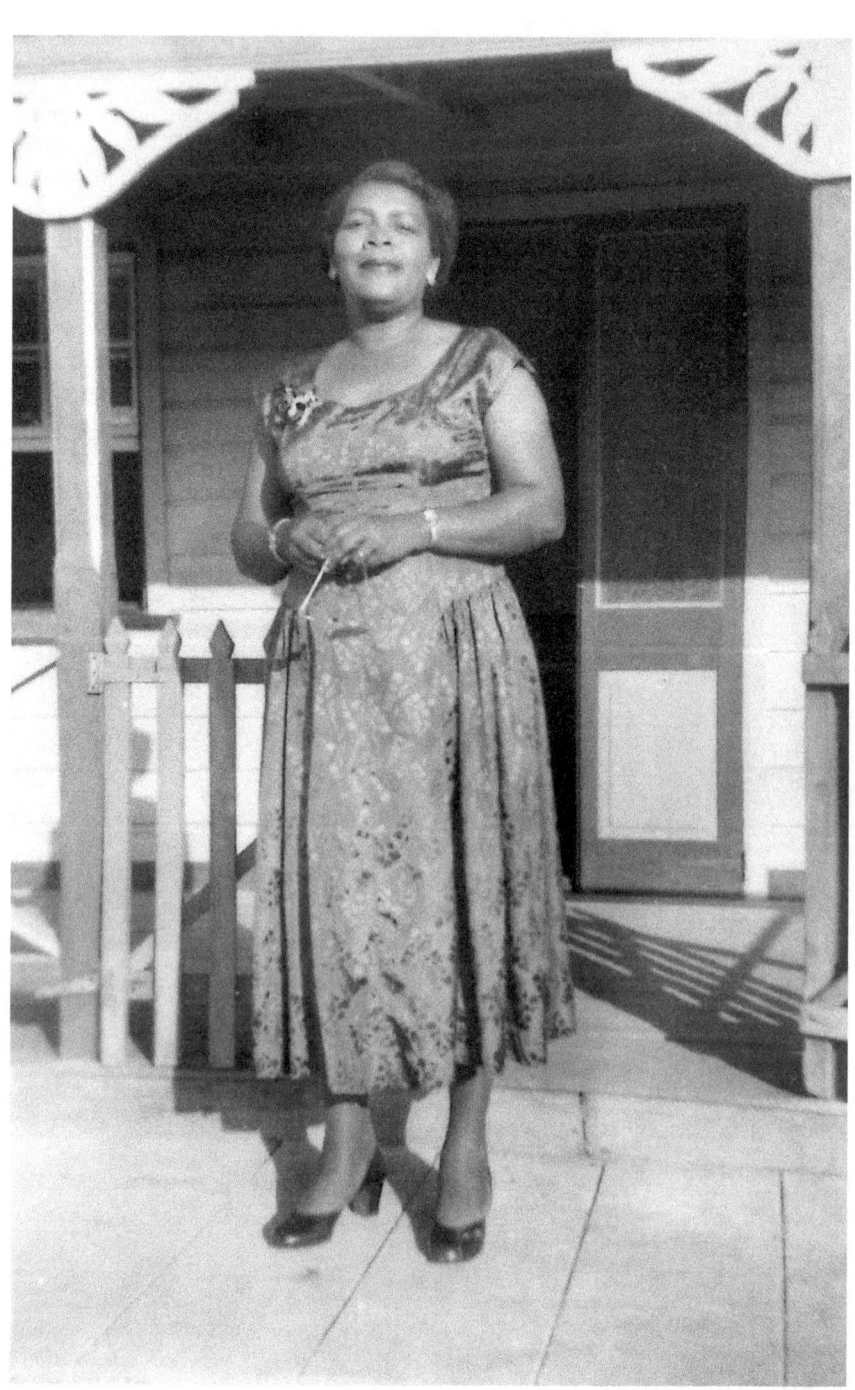

My mother, Eileen Alleyne

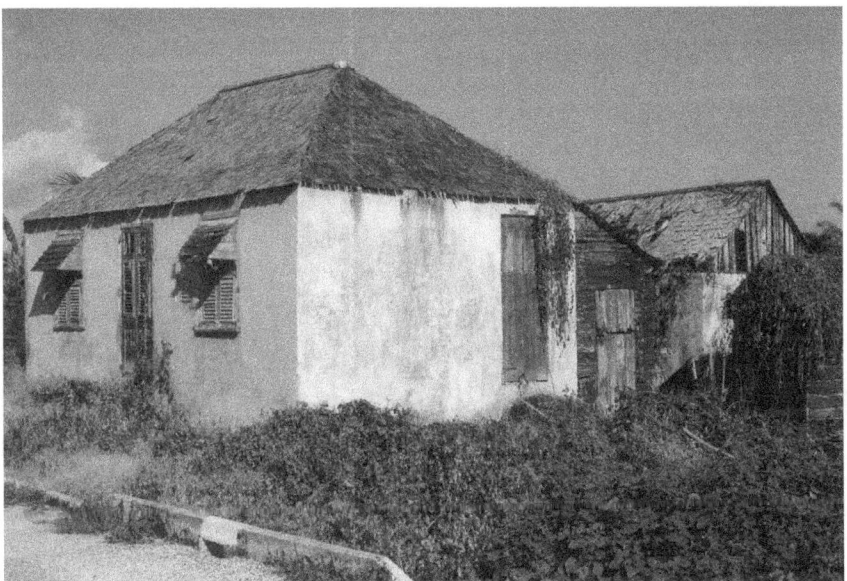

The house where I was born, Lucas Street, St Philip, Barbados

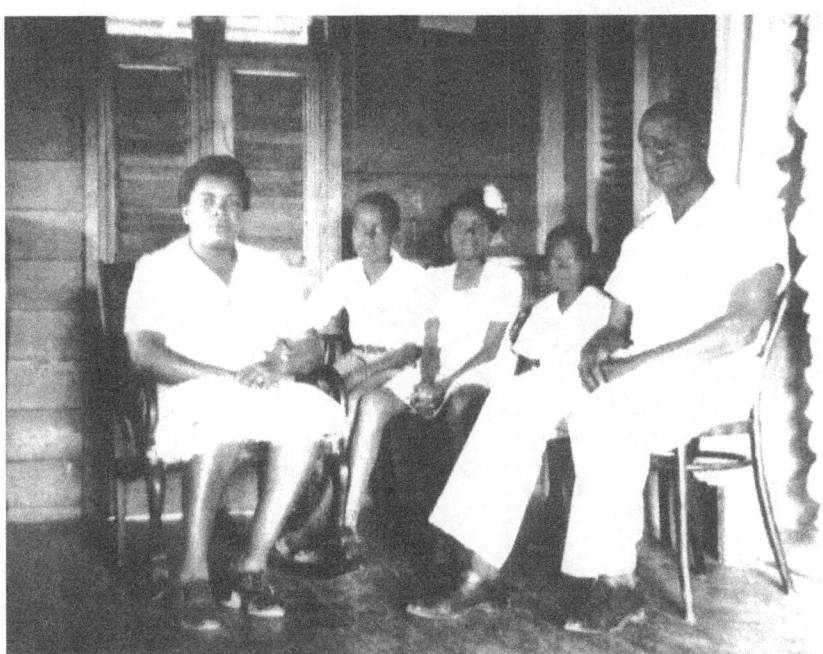

From left to right: My mother, me, my sister Cynthia, my brother Grant, and my father

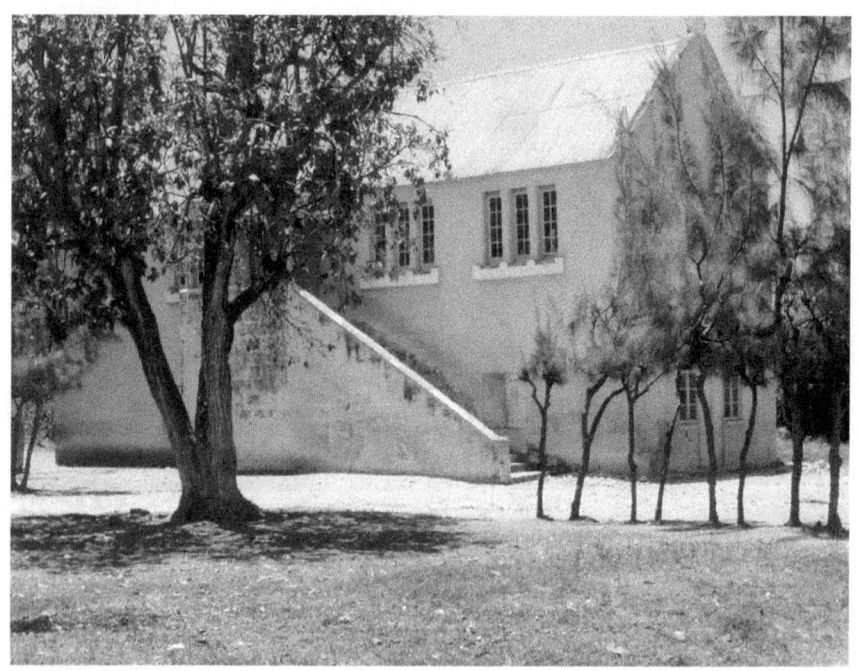

Holy Trinity Elementary School

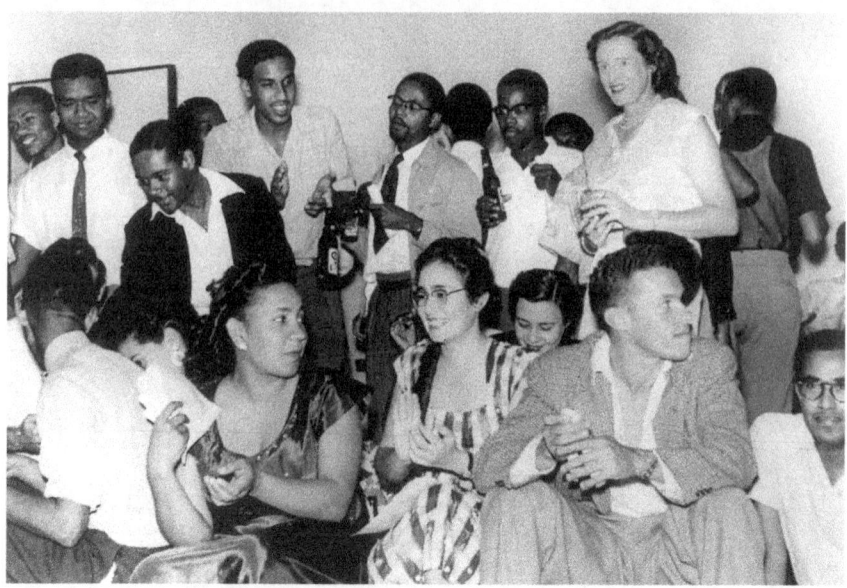

At a medical "smoker" (medical party), 1955 or 1956

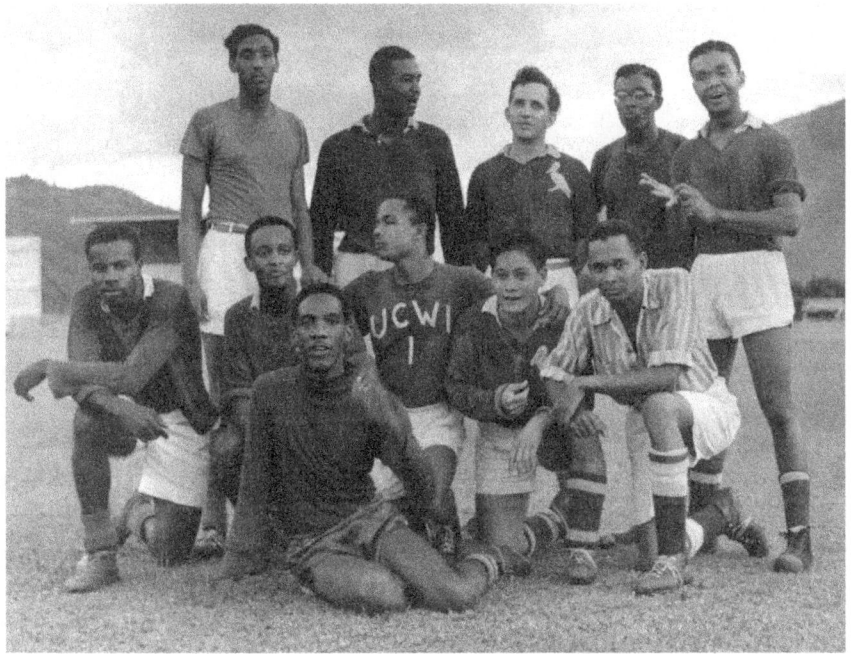

Class of 1957 football team

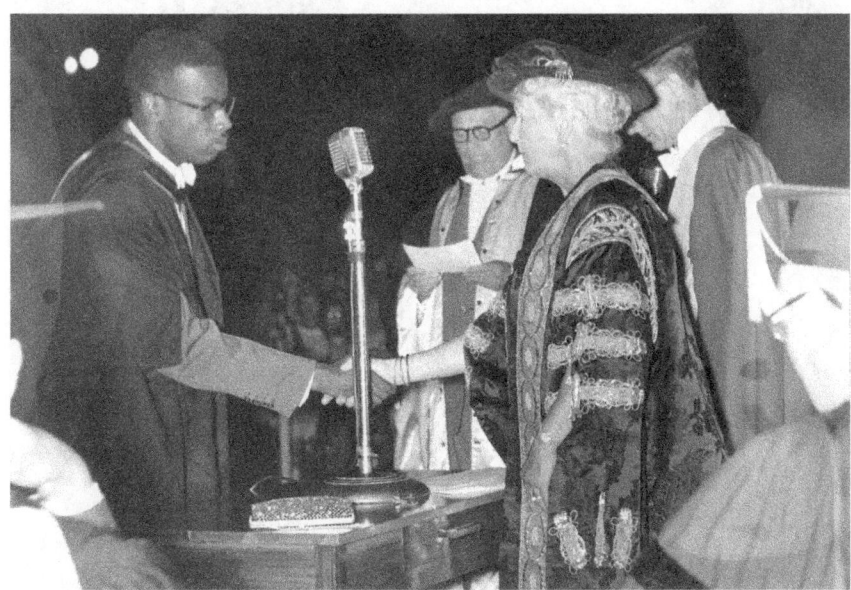

Receiving the MBBS diploma from HRH Princess Alice of Athlone, Chancellor of the University College of the West Indies, 1958

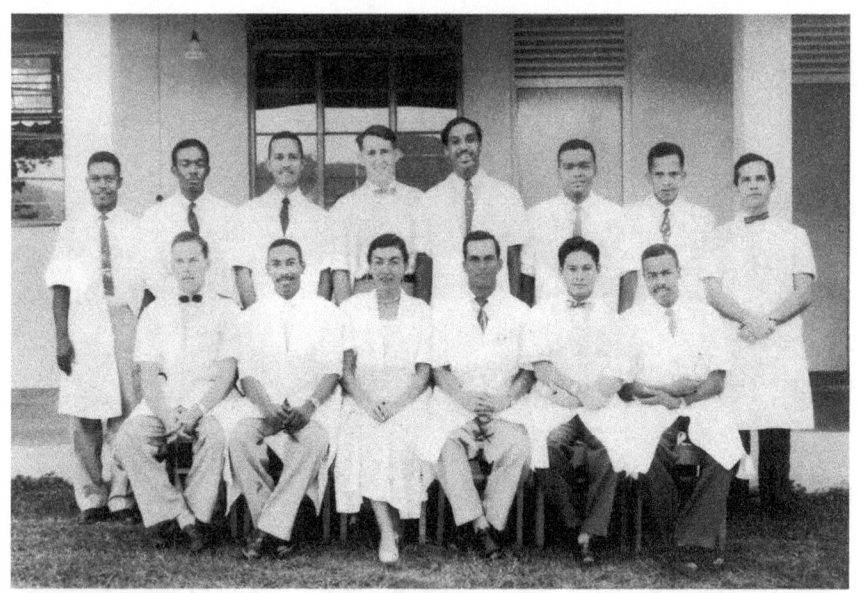

Young colleague doctors, 1958

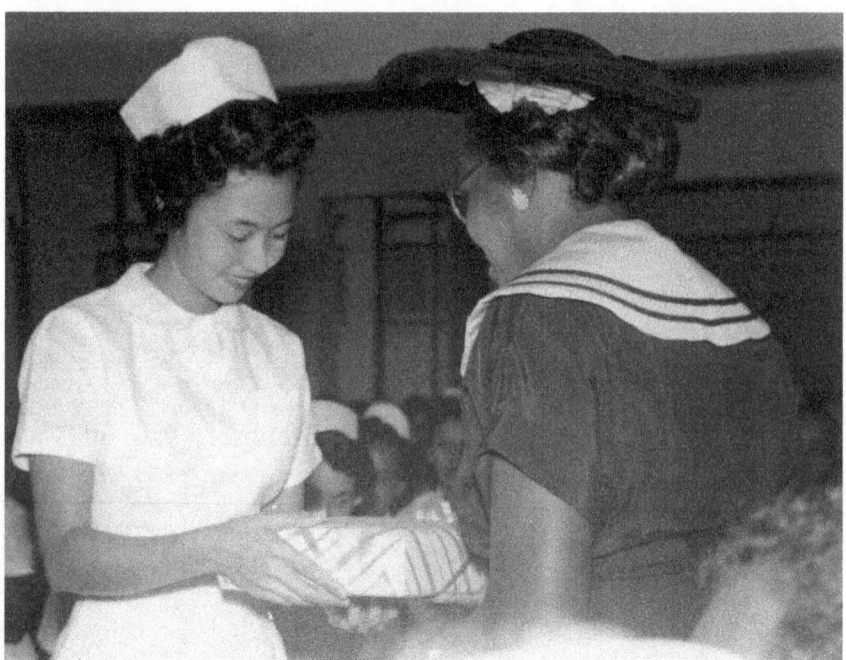

Sylvan with Dame Nita Barrow, University College Hospital's nursing students' graduation, 1957

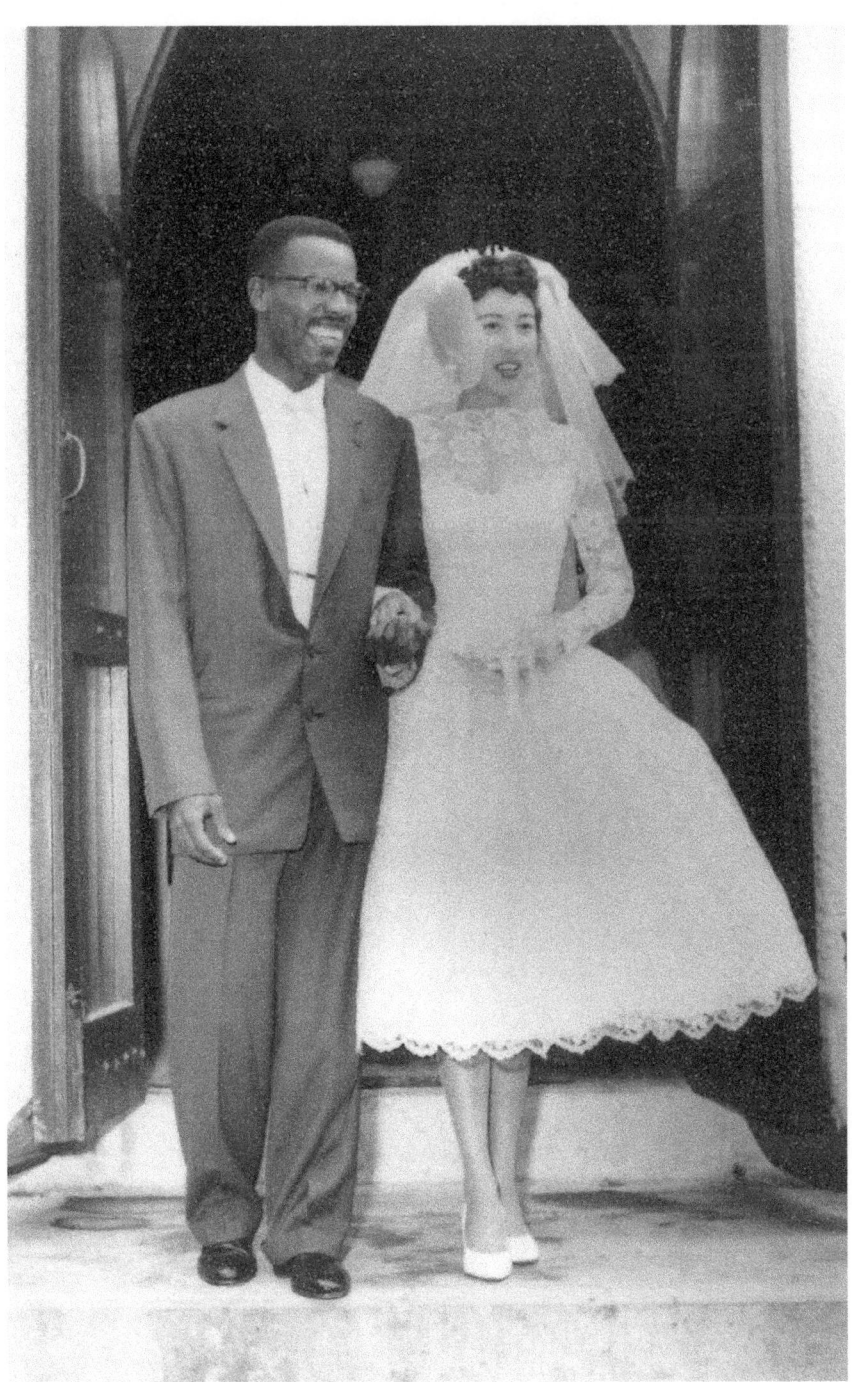

Our wedding, 1958

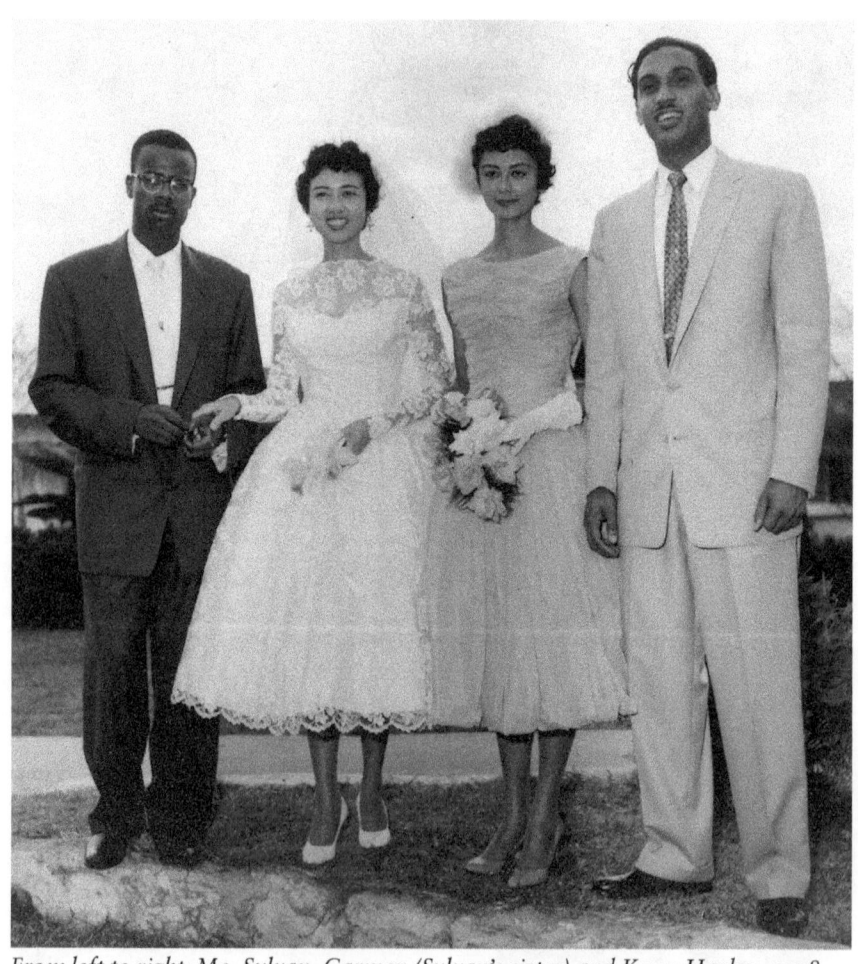
From left to right: Me, Sylvan, Carmen (Sylvan's sister) and Knox Hagley, 1958

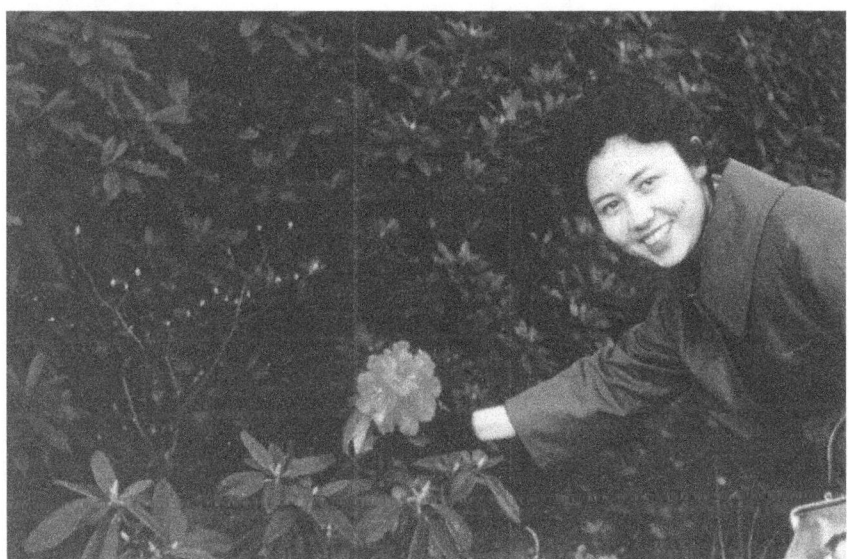

Sylvan with a rhododendron, Kenwood Park, London, England, spring 1962

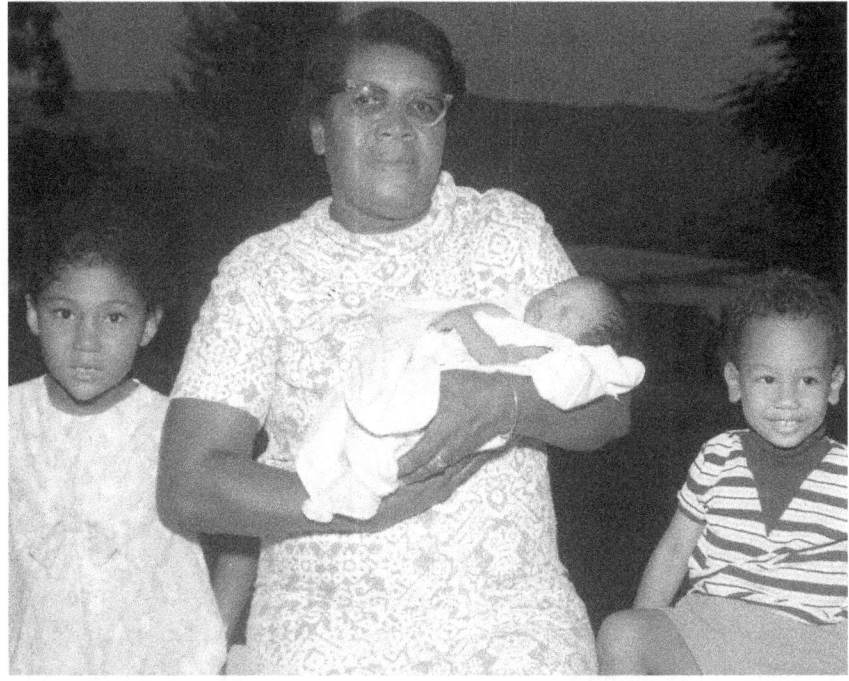

Mama holding Adrian, Carol on one side and Andrew on the other, in Jamaica, c. 1970

CHAPTER 4

My Scientific Career
Sojourn from Clinical Medicine

Before I left Jamaica for New York, Professor Cruickshank had asked what I intended to do next. I could have remained as a registrar, as I was too inexperienced as yet to be a consultant, and in any case, there were no vacancies in the Department of Medicine. I was still thinking of returning to Barbados and in early 1963 had written to the chief medical officer, Dr Byer, to inquire about possible positions in the hospital, where there was a single physician and one medical registrar. The post of registrar was advertised, and I was encouraged to come back to it by Rudolph Daniel, my former teacher and now the government's chief personnel officer. The prospect was that there would in time be a second physician post for which I would then be eligible.

Professor Cruickshank suggested that I see John Waterlow, director of the Tropical Metabolism Research Unit (TMRU), which had been established to study infant malnutrition.[1] John Waterlow had worked in Africa and studied the problem in the West Indies as early as 1945 and eventually was able to persuade the British Medical Research Council to establish a unit in Jamaica in 1956 to study its clinical and physiological aspects. The unit, though in the university, was initially an expatriate enclave with all English staff. It consisted of a metabolic ward and well-equipped laboratories. I went to see John at his flat one Sunday morning, and after a few drinks of rum, he invited me to work in the TMRU. I agreed and then wrote to Dr Byer, asking for an extension of my no-pay leave for one year, as "I will soon be committed to some work which I hope will enable me to get my MD and I am sure you would want me to do that if possible." The leave was granted.

THE TROPICAL METABOLISM RESEARCH UNIT

I started in the TMRU in 1963, and on my first day was received by John Garrow, who was acting head of the unit while John Waterlow was away on sabbatical in London. John Garrow greeted me by asking me what I was going to do, as it was up to me to fashion my research agenda. I indicated that I wished to study the renal function of malnourished children. I developed a detailed proposal, which I sent to Professor Waterlow. He shared it with Professor Rosenheim and an experienced renal physician in his medical unit. These latter were concerned by the scope of the work I was proposing, but John Waterlow was all encouragement. My first knowledge of the work of the TMRU had come from a paper by Roger Smith on total body water in malnourished children some years before, and I recall thinking to myself that I and persons like me could carry out what I considered basic research just as well. So John Garrow's question was a proper challenge. The other West Indian in the TMRU then was David Picou, with whom I would develop a fast friendship. We were both driven and competitive, and the natural result was periods of turbulence in our relationship, but I believe that we never lost respect for each other and can now be pleased with a friendship that survived those periods.

In late 1964, Rudolph Daniel wrote to me again asking for a definitive answer as to whether I planned to return to Barbados, noting that my post had been "kept on the books". He was not sanguine about the possibilities, however, noting that "with average luck we should have a post here of specialist physician available for you", but he went on to say that he was not allowed to fill any of the existing posts. This seemed very uncertain to me, and I had begun to enjoy my work immensely, so reluctantly I wrote and resigned from the Barbados government service in 1964. I gather that I had been kept in the service as a port health officer in order to retain a position and my pension rights. In retrospect, I have to be grateful to both Maurice Byer and Rudolph Daniel for their concern about my future beyond their professional responsibility for the personnel of the public service.

My introduction to research was unusual. The standard approach now, and one which I certainly followed with my research fellows, would be to discuss in detail the protocol to be used and the number of experiments to be carried out, review the background literature and submit a detailed proposal to the institutional review board. There was none of this. John Garrow believed that you should be left to your own devices, and if you were any good, you would swim; if not, you would be frustrated and give up. He would be available for consultation but would never ask to review your results. This meant that I had to design my experiment, find the necessary apparatus, which included borrowing an old infusion pump, and practise the chemical assays myself.

In order to measure renal function, I had to collect timed specimens of urine, so I devised a unique way of determining when the infants urinated. A tube came from a cup fastened around the child's perineum and drained into a beaker on a beam balance. When the child passed urine, the beaker would be depressed, which triggered a bell, enabling the observer to note the time and volume of urine passed. My first attempts were a disaster, until it was pointed out that I had not observed the appropriate relation of the centre of gravity to the fulcrum of the balance. John Garrow's cryptic comment was that if I had spent my time studying something useful such as physics instead of Latin and Greek, I would have appreciated these elementary principles. A colleague remarked once that I was running the risk of instilling a Pavlovian response in these young children. He feared that when they became adults and heard a bell ring, they might be seized by an overwhelming desire to pass urine.

My research prospered. Initially I measured the renal function in malnutrition, as I had proposed, and found, as others had done, that it was impaired and gradually recovered as the children's nutritional state improved. I theorized that this might be the result of cardiac insufficiency and that the swelling which characterized some forms of malnutrition might be an indication that the infants had mild cardiac failure. So I determined to measure the cardiac output in these children and proposed to use a method that involved injecting a dye and measuring its passage through the body. This produced dye-dilution curves from which cardiac output could be calculated. This method had only ever been used in white persons,

My Scientific Career: Sojourn from Clinical Medicine

as it was possible that skin pigment might prevent measurement of the injected dye. The equipment to carry out this measurement was expensive, but when I made the proposal to John Waterlow, he simply said *go ahead* and proceeded to order it. Thankfully it was possible to measure the cardiac output, which was impaired and provided at least one explanation of the diminished renal function. I presented the results of this work for my doctorate of the University of London,[2] and the thesis was accepted without my having to do any revision. My research explored many other aspects of the biochemical and physiological changes that occurred in infantile malnutrition in addition to the disturbance of renal and cardiac function.

My work, which often involved finding ingenious solutions to problems, convinced me of my own capacity to overcome difficulties which might appear insuperable, and instilled or rather strengthened a self-confidence at which I sometimes marvel. When we did not have needed equipment, we simply made it. When I visit laboratories today and see commercial constriction micropipettes being discarded, I cringe as I recall learning to make my own from glass tubing.

I witnessed the beginning of a line of work that has had enormous impact on thinking about early childhood development and the permanence of changes due to malnutrition. One of my students, Herbert Ho Ping Kong, remarked one morning that it was inappropriate to have children restrained in cots during experiments and also to have them remain confined in the intervals between experiments while they were recovering or had recovered. It was agreed that play should be an essential part of the recovery, and a playpen was constructed in the metabolic ward. Eventually a physician interested in development psychology, Sally McGregor, came to the unit and continued and expanded this work, demonstrating conclusively the effect of play and stimulation on the recovery of cognitive function after an episode of malnutrition. Subsequent studies on the long-term effects of malnutrition have demonstrated that malnourished children suffer from stunted growth. It has also been shown that stunting in children leads to intellectual impairment as well as subsequent antisocial behaviours.

But in addition, I learned to appreciate some of the history of science and the philosophical concepts that drove experimentation. I was entranced by the writings of Karl Popper[3] and took almost instinctively to the hypothetical deductive approach. I was chastened by his thesis that falsification is the normal fate of all hypotheses, and there would come a day when my carefully elaborated hypotheses would be shown to be inadequate by further explication of the natural phenomena, aided no doubt by more powerful technology. On reflection now, I appreciate that this must be the cause of some of the liberating exhilaration of science. At the time, I read and reread Peter Medawar's *Advice to a Young Scientist*[4] as well as some of his other works. More recently I have found it salutary to read again some of this work from a distance of fifty years and reflect on its relevance to my decision to work in a scientific institution for seven years and be so thoroughly engrossed in it. There must have been some inquisitiveness – a desire to understand the nature of the physiological changes that caused clinical signs and symptoms. Medawar comforted and stimulated me when he wrote in *Advice to a Young Scientist*, "Whatever the motives that persuade anyone to pursue a career in scientific research, a scientist must very much want to be one. In my anxiety that they should not be underestimated, I may sometimes make too much of the vexations and frustrations of scientific life, but it can be one of great contentment and reward (I do not mean, although I do not exclude, material reward), with the added satisfaction of using one's energies to the full."

There was perhaps a small dose of arrogance. There must have been the feeling that I, or rather we West Indians, could be as good at research and explaining clinical phenomena as other persons. We could publish in the same prestigious journals as others. My early work was entirely clinical research and not experimentation, in the sense that I introduced some external agent to change the system and measured the nature and size of the change. The only differences I measured were those that occurred as a result of malnutrition itself and those occurring during the recovery phase. In later work on animals, I would induce metabolic changes and measure the effect of the change on various organ systems.

There must have been a considerable degree of competitiveness and the wish to be the first to describe one or other phenomenon. In this sense, one method of keeping score of one's achievements was tracking the number of publications produced. Priority is important to scientists, and perhaps the main thing a scientist can really own is the knowledge of pre-eminence

My Scientific Career: Sojourn from Clinical Medicine

and recognition of priority of his findings. Over time I would appreciate that Peter Medawar's advice on research being the art of the soluble really meant that research had to look for those aspects of the problem that could be addressed, given the available knowledge and technology.[5] Of course, this goes along with the hubristic attitude that all scientific problems are eventually soluble.

I carried out a considerable body of research on animals, which was stimulated initially by the time I spent in 1967 on a sabbatical in Boston University in the laboratory of Dr Arnold Relman, a distinguished nephrologist and an introduction to renal biochemistry. Living in Boston was also a stimulating experience. I was met and entertained by a delightful rogue of a cousin, Bindley Wilshire. We lived in a small apartment in Brookline, a predominantly Jewish part of Boston, and Sylvan and I look back on those days and the friends we made with much pleasure. We met several West Indians or persons with West Indian connections and were accepted into many American homes for enjoyable social gatherings. This was during the Vietnam War, and the palpable loneliness of some new wives whose husbands were fighting there often provoked discussion on the uselessness of such conflicts. We visited some of the delightful small towns around Boston, including Plymouth, that historic site of the disembarkation of the Mayflower pilgrims.

There were three other fellows working in the laboratory on different aspects of renal intermediary metabolism. This meant I had to read and learn the biochemistry to which I had paid scant attention in medical school, and I found myself engaged in friendly competition with my colleagues. I learned a tremendous amount both technically and clinically and was driven to read the scientific literature even more voraciously, as it was almost unforgivable not to have read a paper on some aspect of kidney function which my colleagues had read. This competition, very much a part of the Americans' scientific culture, was new to me, but before long I found myself immersed in it.

It had been known for some time that when mammals took a substance that made the blood more acid, the kidneys excreted ammonia derived principally from the amino acid glutamine.[6] And in addition to excreting ammonia, the kidneys made glucose, a process known as gluconeogenesis.[7]

In Boston I participated in experiments that attempted to show that the same phenomenon occurred in dogs. It was not clear, however, how the metabolic process was controlled, and I returned to Jamaica with the idea that a specific enzyme was responsible.

My colleagues and I in Jamaica could confirm that ammonia and glucose production were indeed linked. The time sequence of the response to an acid load and the consequent metabolic changes in the kidney were the subject of a long line of research. We discovered the nature of the critical enzymatic response that led to increased glucose production by the kidney and carried out several experiments around the consequent changes in renal biochemistry. We would detail the characteristics of the enzyme and its location in the kidney cell as well as the changes in other organs and their control. One of our more significant findings was that there was a specific factor in the plasma of the acidotic rats that stimulated the biochemical changes in the kidney.[8]

Many years later, I was saved from an embarrassing situation when at the beginning of a formal lecture in Ireland on my research, the carousel with all my slides fell, and I was forced to fill in the time. I spoke about the origin of the word *ammonia*. I could tell the audience that it derives from the odour around the temple of Jupiter Ammon, which was caused by the camels urinating in the surrounding sand. I think the anecdote remained with them long after they had forgotten my information about renal metabolism.

I was fortunate to have excellent collaborators in this work. These included Hernando Flores, a visiting Chilean biochemist; Ann Roobol, a British biochemist; and Harvey Besterman and George Scullard, British medical students who were spending a year in the unit. There was also excellent technical help. It is still somewhat amazing to recall the sophistication of the research carried out, comparable with that from any laboratory in the world, and we were recognized as being one of the world's leading groups on this aspect of renal metabolism.[9]

My initial research on the renal and cardiac function in malnutrition expanded to involve studies on body composition, hormonal metabolism and other metabolic disturbances in the malnourished child. Much of the emphasis in the studies on body composition was around the metabolism of

My Scientific Career: Sojourn from Clinical Medicine

potassium, an important ion for many body processes. The malnourished child is deficient in potassium, and it was possible to elaborate and prove a theory that deficiency could be as a result of the capacity of the body tissues, mainly muscle, to retain potassium, or it could be that the content of potassium in these tissues was low. In severe malnutrition it was probably a combination of both and as the child recovered not only did the capacity or muscle mass increase, but it acquired its proper concentration of potassium. We also conducted seminal studies of other aspects of renal function, carbohydrate metabolism and the hormonal response to malnutrition.

I was particularly pleased to be able to attract some young West Indian men to work with me for shorter or longer periods, and some of them have become prestigious academics. Herbert Ho Ping Kong, now a distinguished physician in Toronto, Canada, carried out work on sickle-cell crises for his PhD thesis. Wendell Wilson also studied renal function in sickle-cell anaemia for his doctorate, and Henry Fraser, who spent an elective with me, subsequently became professor of medicine and dean of the faculty. TMRU was a hive of activity, and the atmosphere was ideal for the development of young scientists. Our internal seminars, at which we presented our work, often in progress, were spectacular for the range and depth of the topics covered and were attended by many from other parts of the university. The intellectual jousting, the collegiality, the constant discussion of one's data and opining on those of colleagues were extraordinary experiences. Along with several remarkable colleagues, we were able to make several seminal scientific observations resulting in a high rate of publication in prestigious scientific journals. The culture of self-experimentation produced some humorous examples of the extremes to which we went.

One of these resulted from experiments I was carrying out which were outside the mainstream of my work in malnutrition. I was measuring the impact of a diuretic triamterene, which was being proposed as an alternative to thiazide diuretics, because unlike thiazides, it did not produce a fall in plasma potassium. Diuretics were and are a standard agent in the treatment of hypertension. The only small inconvenience was that some metabolite of triamterene caused urine to fluoresce in the dark. One of my colleagues volunteered to take the drug, and on coming home late one night and going to the bathroom, he did not turn on the light for fear of disturbing his wife. One can imagine the consternation at the appearance of this bright fluorescent stream. The lesson is that one should alert one's experimental subjects in advance about the possible complications.

I travelled frequently to scientific meetings, but one of the more memorable trips was at the invitation from the International Pediatric Association to be part of a group of young physicians from developing countries to visit the Scandinavian countries. The group included two women from the Dominican Republic and the Philippines, and men from Thailand, Nigeria, Tanzania and three others. We attended seminars and gave interviews in Finland, Sweden, Norway and Denmark, and then we went on to Vienna for the International Pediatric Conference. The group bonded easily, and the commonality of the colonial experience was obvious to all of us. The other striking feature was the emphasis we all had on clinical skills. I was not a paediatrician, and yet my major contribution was in paediatric nutrition, and I could speak authoritatively about childhood malnutrition and several aspects of its pathophysiology.

I was invited by a young Norwegian paediatrician to their family home one weekend, where I had a sauna for the first time. The experience of running from the sauna and jumping into an icy cold lake is one I can never forget. I thought my heart had stopped.

After six weeks we ended up in Vienna at the congress, where I was invited to participate in a pre-congress conference. I had rarely been more frustrated. Though I had prepared the various topics well, I noted that my pertinent interventions were virtually ignored, while to my mind, the less accurate pontifications of the great old men were listened to with rapt attention.

On leaving the conference hall, however, I was amazed to meet on the street Wilfred Cartey, who had been at university with me – in fact, his room at one time was next to mine. Years earlier, he had come from Trinidad and Tobago to Jamaica in a plane, which of course was not pressurized, and he suffered what was eventually diagnosed as a painful sickle-cell crisis. He went on to become an accomplished author, and one day, while writing a letter sitting in a plane, he suddenly went blind, presumably due to blocked retinal arteries. He was now a professor of African studies at Columbia University in New York. He recognized my voice when I hailed

My Scientific Career: Sojourn from Clinical Medicine

him, and we spent a few glorious days and nights in Vienna. Interestingly, his travelling companions were always beautiful young women, but I never got a clear answer from him as to how he chose them or, rather, how they chose him. My most vivid memories are of the heurigens, where, in the wee hours of the morning, we would sing calypsos, and the German patrons would sing their songs. Wine is a great leveller.

Work in Jamaica presented certain challenges. In Boston, for example, we had used liquid nitrogen to fast-freeze tissues, but in Jamaica, we had only a liquid air machine, so we used liquid air instead. Measurement of a certain metabolite in the rat kidney could be done only with an enzyme that was not only expensive but also scarce, though it could be extracted from the muscle of a particular worm. So I went to Puerto Rico, visited an abattoir, and came back to Jamaica with my thermos full of worms, from which I extracted the required enzyme. Our rats, which were used in all our research on renal metabolism, were from a strain imported from the United States and fed with imported rat chow. Some official in one of the ministries of government decided that there was nothing special about rat chow and that it could easily be manufactured locally, so we were denied an import licence and were forced to feed our rats on the locally produced chow. After about two weeks, our rats became completely bald. We made representation to the appropriate government department, and fortunately, on the basis of the evidence, our import licence was renewed. Of course, we had to sacrifice the bald rats and begin a new colony with imported rats. A colleague suggested that if I could establish the missing ingredient in the local chow, and if it could be shown that that ingredient could restore hair to bald men, our unit could become rich.

When my experiments called for feeding my rats in the evening, after I'd gone home, I would have to return to the laboratory to feed them and on occasion would take my little daughter with me. One afternoon at a children's party, they were speaking about what work their fathers did. When it came to my six-year-old daughter's turn, she said proudly, "My daddy feeds rats."

On several occasions, especially at international meetings, when I would explain puckishly that I worked in Jamaica – not Jamaica, Long Island, but the Jamaica that was ninety miles south of Cuba – I had cause to reflect on the possibilities and difficulties of research in developing countries. I would say to my colleagues in Boston that there was no special geographical predilection in terms of distribution of talent or ideas. The difficulty was that we in the developing world, because of technological problems and deficient facilities, had to be much more resourceful. This was often part of the debate as to whether scientists from developing countries should concentrate only on the science leading to solutions of domestic problems or should also enter the lists with scientists from other parts of the world and try to solve problems common to humanity. I addressed this in the lecture I gave in Barbados in 1978 on medical research in the Caribbean.[10]

> I would like, however, to think that our medical scientists in their quest for excellence are regarding themselves as scientists from the Caribbean and not narrowly as Caribbean scientists. It is not a semantic differential. In this matter I agree with Sir Arthur Lewis, who advises us to sidestep our cultural nationalists, for whom our own thing is always better than other people's things, and I hope we do not develop a scientific counterpart of the ethnocentricity of the developmental sociologists.

Of course, it is argued that this applies only to the physical sciences and the efforts to unravel the secrets of nature. This dichotomy is much less obvious in the social sciences. There are aspects of life and living and of the adaptation of mankind to the local environment that lend themselves uniquely to local study, which is not inhibited by lack of technology. My observations are also more relevant to the narrow field of medical science and research and do not touch the much broader issue of science and technology as a spur to the economic growth of countries. This is perhaps addressed best with relationship to the role of universities and tertiary level institutions.

I should describe Sylvan's work here. While we were in Barbados preparing to go to London, she was convinced by one of our friends that she should study for the certificate in social work at the London School of Economics. She was accepted in 1963 but decided to return to Jamaica with me instead. She then entered the University College of the West Indies, completed her certificate and then her BSc in social work, and worked as a research fellow in the Department of Social and Preventive Medicine. She was subsequently appointed a lecturer in social work in the Department of Sociology and carried out a number of research studies predominantly on the social aspects of chronic disease. She was exempted from the master's degree on the basis of her published work and allowed to proceed to work for her PhD, which she eventually obtained in 1987. While working on her PhD, she completed the master's degree in social work from Catholic University in Maryland.

SCIENTIFIC SECRETARY, COMMONWEALTH CARIBBEAN MEDICAL RESEARCH COUNCIL

I was one of the scientific secretaries of the Commonwealth Caribbean Medical Research Council from 1969 to 1981, when I left the university. This council represented the unbroken continuation of Caribbean-wide support for research that had its origins in post–Second World War colonial interest in research and development. After the war, a colonial medical research committee in Britain advised the Colonial Office on stimulating research and provided funding for research committees such as had been formed in Africa in 1952. A similar committee was established in the West Indies in 1956 with great fanfare, including speeches by Norman Manley, then chief minister of Jamaica. The committee was named the Scientific Advisory Committee and theoretically advised the secretary of state for the colonies on the state of research in the Caribbean. As a senior medical student, I attended the first scientific meeting that accompanied the formal opening, and I have vivid memories of some of the more engaging presentations. An obstetrician, Dr J. Parboosingh, presented a case of "Unusual Bleeding Associated with Pregnancy" and described pint by pint the numerous blood transfusions that were employed to save the life of his patient.

John Waterlow was the first secretary, and with the advent of the West Indies Federation in 1960, he proposed that the committee become a Caribbean Medical Research Council. The federation dissolved in 1962, but it was not until 1972 that the Scientific Advisory Committee was converted into the Commonwealth Caribbean Medical Research Council. Like the Scientific Advisory Committee, the council had as its two main functions administration of small research grants and the organization of research meetings. John Waterlow was succeeded as scientific secretary by John Garrow, then David Picou, myself and Errol Waldron. The council has changed its name to the Caribbean Health Research Council, and its annual research meetings are still the primary events of this nature in the Caribbean. One of the functions of the scientific secretaries was to visit the several Caribbean countries prior to the annual meetings to solicit contributions for the programme, and some of these visits stand out for the opportunity they presented to see how medical services were organized and the conditions under which research was carried out. Most of the contributions came from the medical faculty of the university, but there were also significant, mainly clinical presentations from general practitioners and doctors working in the government services. The meetings were held in various countries and were marked not only by the splendid scientific presentations but also social events which the countries vied in arranging.

One of my more memorable visits was to Guyana in 1968, when I visited Dr George Giglioli, whom I had heard speak at the first meeting of the council in 1956. He is still recognized as one of the finest public health researchers who ever worked in the Caribbean. He had been the first person to employ DDT in the Caribbean and had made the coastal area of Guyana (then British Guiana) free of malaria. He received me kindly on his veranda, and we spoke initially about the forthcoming meeting of the research council and whether he was continuing research and would think of presenting a paper. He declined to participate and then asked me what I was doing – what was my job? I spoke about my research in the TMRU and the pleasure I derived from clinical investigation. He then quietly asked me about my family – what were the occupations of my parents, and how were my siblings faring? When I told him of my origins, he enquired why I was interested in an academic life rather than, as he put it, "securing my financial future". He spoke also about advising young Guyanese to secure their financial futures so that their children could be spared the economic hardships their parents had had to undergo. I confess that I bridled a bit and wondered why this man, recognized and lauded for dedicating his life to public health and research, should dissuade a young Caribbean investigator. Was it because he thought good research beyond us? So I asked him pointedly why he had chosen his career and dedicated himself to public health and research in a place like Guyana. He told me that his father had been a professor of anatomy, and sundry relatives had been distinguished university academics, so it was natural for him to follow a path which in his view was an anomaly for me. Out of respect I did not continue the discussion, but I wondered how Caribbean children would become academics and try to increase the store of knowledge if there were no antecedents and models for them to follow.

He gave me a book he had written on malarial nephritis, which had been published in 1932[11] – the year I was born. I subsequently acquired a cyclostyled copy of his personal autobiography entitled *Demerara Doctor: An Early Success against Malaria*,[12] and John Waterlow and I persuaded the Rockefeller Foundation to provide a grant to the London School of Hygiene and Tropical Medicine for its publication. The book contains a fascinating account of his life in meticulous detail, and one has to marvel at the careful, extensive notes he must have kept. He describes how one of his jobs was to be the medical officer in a bauxite mine, where he noticed that hookworm infection was prevalent. Indeed, sixty-eight per cent of the workers were infected because of the poor sanitation and the fact that few wore shoes. He carried out mass treatment of the workers with carbon tetrachloride over a four-day period. Of interest is a letter written to him subsequently by the manager. Two of its paragraphs read as follows:

> In the beginning of 1923 96 miners on the ore face were mining 342 tons of bauxite per working day, whereas on 1 February 1924 76 miners at the ore face are mining 540 tons of bauxite per working day.
>
> I cannot say I attribute this increase in the output of ore per man per day entirely to the treatment which you gave for hookworm, but I do think that, to a great extent, the elimination of this disease has had something to do with our increased output and our reduction of costs. For the five months previous to September 1923 the increase in tonnage per man per day was nil, whereas during the five months following September 1923, hour increase in tonnage has amounted to one and three-quarter tons per man per day.

Unfortunately, it was subsequently discovered that carbon tetrachloride was damaging to the liver, but apparently Dr Giglioli had found no toxic complications.

JOHN WATERLOW THE MAGNANIMOUS

John was remarkable in many ways and not only as a scientist. His trust was almost simplistic, and he would go to enormous lengths to support those in whom he believed. I am still touched today by reading his letters to the Medical Research Council agitating for better salaries for David Picou and myself, who were being paid on scales and rates lower than those of the expatriate staff. He even offered to supplement our salaries from his pocket – which, of course, we declined. I cite one example of his magnanimity.

In 1969, Sylvan and I adopted a baby girl, Carol, and I began to think that it was about time I bought a house. I learned that John Hayes in the university's pathology department was going to Boston and that his house was for sale. I went along and said to John, "I hear you are selling your house. How much are you asking for it?" To which John replied, "Six thousand pounds." I then said, "Okay, I will buy it." We shook hands and that was that.

Immediately after that conversation, I was walking into the unit, and John Waterlow saw me looking preoccupied. I told him that I had just agreed to buy a house, and I would now have to look for the money, at which he offered immediately to lend me three thousand pounds, which he did without any formal note. I duly paid John Hayes three thousand pounds and while the lawyers were arranging the formalities, he left for Boston with the assurance that my word was good for the remaining money. Some months later, John Waterlow suggested that I give him an IOU for the three thousand pounds he had lent me, which I did. About two years later, I paid him, and he returned the cancelled IOU. Twenty-five years later, I got a note from him which said that he had been putting his papers in order and noticed that he had lent me three thousand pounds but could not find any record of my having repaid him. The letter concluded thus: "If indeed you did not repay me, don't worry about it now." Luckily I had kept the cancelled IOU and could send him a copy, to which he replied, "You need not have bothered."

John's concern about the welfare of his staff was perhaps a mixture of paternal instinct and a natural desire to protect his turf. He took considerable pride in the scientific development of David Picou and myself, as we

My Scientific Career: Sojourn from Clinical Medicine

justified his contention that there were West Indians capable of good science and being leaders in their fields. This was contrary to the philosophy of the Medical Research Council, which was essentially colonial in outlook. There were Medical Research Council units in Africa which where run exclusively by expatriates with no African scientists on staff. Thus John was wary of others trying to poach on his domain and steal away his chickens. I was never fully aware of the depth of this feeling until I was brought up against it on one occasion in about 1969.

John was persuaded that we should mount an Open Day as one mechanism of making our work better known in the university and possibly attracting young graduates to come and work in the unit. The Caribbean Food and Nutrition Institute was a sister, or rival, unit also situated on the university campus. It had arisen out of concern for the public health aspect of nutrition and was headed by Dick Jelliffe, who had been the first head of paediatrics in the university but left to develop considerable expertise in the public health aspects of nutrition. The institute was supported by international foundations and eventually by the Pan American Health Organization (PAHO). Dick came to our Open Day, and as I was showing him some of the data from my research, he discreetly suggested that I come and work with him. He proposed that I go to the United States for a master's degree in public health with a focus on nutrition, and on my return, he could almost promise that I would eventually replace him as director of the institute. I remember clearly his ending the proposition saying, "And now that I have sown the seed of a more useful career in your life, I will steal quietly away." I thanked him but gave it little more thought, as the prospect of the work and path he had proposed seemed unattractive. Sometime later I mentioned the incident casually to John, and I had never seen him so furious. He even threatened to go and "have it out" with Dick Jelliffe. I do not know if he was mollified even by my assuring him that I had no intention of taking up the offer.

I tried to capture some of the spirit of those days in TMRU in a speech I gave after dinner at the Royal College of Physicians to honour John Waterlow at his eightieth birthday festschrift. It was entitled "The Houses that John Built", and I still regard it as one of my finest. I opened this way:

It is an honour to have been asked to give this tribute to John Waterlow – and I intend to use one of the pristine meanings of the word tribute, as something of value given as a token of loyalty or esteem from lieges to their lord. In days of old men paid tribute in specie and spices, in precious stones or the bounty of the land. Silver and gold have we none, but what we bring to you as a tribute this evening, John, are our appreciation of what you have done and our admiration of what you are – all etched and framed in the recollection of personal experiences.

I will pretend that I have returned to ancestral roots and am an ancient griot and will tell some of the stories of your prowess and your interactions with us, with the security that our tradition of oral history stitches the true and meaningful tapestry of the past.

I described the intellectual foundations of his first house, the TMRU, and how he had moved to London to build another, and the legends he had created in his time. I described the legend of the master and his prodigious scientific output to prove it. He was, I said,

the skilled craftsman with a respected place in the guild of his peers – true scientists. He imbued large numbers of us with a love for scientific enquiry, to follow what we took to be the truth, always with the belief that the nutritional sciences were one of the true basic sciences and when we encountered difficulties – *solvitur ambulando!* – a sentiment that was clearly appreciated by Bob Marley when he advised us not to worry because – *every little thing will be all right*!

I described his impatience with the artificial separation of research: "He used to say, there are only two kinds of research – good and bad. In the true tradition of the master he let his apprentices grow and he believed that "he serves his master ill who remains a pupil still". As a master and genuine leader, John displayed and displays perhaps the most important quality of a leader – the leader listens." I emphasized his benevolence. He was kindness personified to many of us, helping distinguished scientists, maids and messengers, gardeners and guards.

I ended by saying of him what Jane Addams said of George Washington: "The lessons of great men are lost unless they reinforce upon our minds the highest demands which we make upon ourselves – they are lost unless they drive our sluggish wills forward in the direction of their highest ideals."

John Waterlow returned to Britain in 1970 to a chair in human nutrition in the London School of Hygiene and Tropical Medicine and established another nutrition unit. He would say later that he felt comfortable leaving Jamaica, as there were West Indians capable of continuing the work. He was succeeded by David Picou, who did ensure the continuation of the tradition of excellence in research. John died in 2010, and at a memorial service, I referred to him in the terms of Virgil's hero: "the arms of creativity, conviction, commitment and compassion borne by one who is a hero to many of us here. John Waterlow".

Little did I know, my career was about to take a dramatic turn.

CHAPTER 5

The Professor of Medicine
My Appointment

While working in the Tropical Metabolism Research Unit, I had maintained contact with clinical medicine and, along with Eugene Ward, professor of physiology, ran a nephrology clinic in the University Hospital of the West Indies. In late 1971, Professor Eric Cruickshank told me that he was leaving and encouraged me to apply for his chair in medicine. I was naturally pleased to be encouraged and made all arrangements to submit an application, which I did formally on 20 January 1972. I named as my referees John Waterlow, Sir Max Rosenheim, my former professor at University College, London, and Sir Harold Himsworth. The last was a former secretary of the UK Medical Research Council who had visited the TMRU on several occasions and knew of my work. Then I received a letter from John Waterlow indicating that the Medical Research Council wished to consider me for the position of director of the Dunn Nutritional Laboratory in Cambridge. The Dunn was then the most prestigious Medical Research Council nutrition unit in the United Kingdom and was headed by Dr Ernest Kodicek, who had established an international reputation for his and the laboratory's work on Vitamin A. The council wished the laboratory, as they put it, to be closely concerned with practical nutritional problems of public health in the United Kingdom and in developing countries. The council was seeking applicants with research experience in the nutritional sciences and preferred to appoint a director with a medical qualification. Incidentally the salary was of the order of five thousand

The Professor of Medicine: My Appointment

pounds annually, which was more than twice that of the professor of medicine at Mona – ten thousand Jamaican dollars. This posed a quandary.

Professor Rosenheim wrote to me in January 1972, and his letter opened as follows:

> Dear Champ,
>
> You seem to be a popular young man, as I understand that the MRC is about to advertise for a new Director of the Dunn nutrition laboratory in Cambridge and that your name has been suggested as someone who might be interested. Dr Kodicek who is the present director is retiring shortly. I was rung up by someone at the MRC who wanted to know a bit more about you and I expressed my firm hope that you would stay in Jamaica and get the Medical School ticking over and improving. I realize that when you hear from the MRC or are faced with the advertisement you are going to be put into another quandary and if you would like to write to me and discuss things, please do not hesitate to do so. I do not wish to persuade you one way or the other.

Given the opening gambit, I was amused at the last sentence.

On the other hand, my good friend Sir Hugh Springer, one of the founding fathers of the university, its first registrar, and subsequent governor general of Barbados and one of its national heroes, wrote to me in February 1972. His letter was as follows:

> Dear Champ,
>
> While lunching with John Waterlow today I learned from him that you had been invited to apply for the headship of the MRC unit at Cambridge and that he had the impression that you were hesitating because you also put in for the chair advertised in the Department of Medicine at Mona. I hope you do not mind my writing to you to encourage you to apply for the Cambridge post. I think such an appointment would be good not only for you but also for the UWI and the West Indies. I imagine that you would be happier and more productive there then you would be in a chair at Mona in the immediate future.

I was interviewed for the professorship and received a formal offer of appointment on 16 March 1972. In a letter dated 15 March 1972, the secretary of the Medical Research Council arranged for me to visit the Dunn and be interviewed on 28 March in London. I visited the laboratory, which was an attractive place, not only because of the Cambridge atmosphere, but also because of the availability of the kinds of resources – human, material and financial – which were the dream of a forty-year-old clinical investigator.

I was interviewed at the Medical Research Council, and it went well. At one point when I was asked about my research and its possible relevance to the nutritional problems in the United Kingdom and the developing countries and whether I could adapt to it, Sir Douglas Black, a distinguished nephrologist who would become president of the Royal College of Physicians, interjected before I could reply, saying, "Of course he can. Nephrologists are very capable chaps; they can do anything." This provoked much laughter. At the end of the interview, I repaired to that place in which many decisions are made or confirmed, the men's room, where I was joined by Dr Henry Bunje, secretary of the council, who was enthusiastic about my interview, and who, although he could not offer me the job, made it clear that the committee was impressed and that he hoped I would take the post if and when offered.

I returned to Jamaica at the end of the first week of April 1972 and spent many anxious hours debating with Sylvan whether or not we should go to Cambridge. This obviously was the most important professional decision we had had to make to date. There were the domestic issues, the financial attractions, the possibilities of international reach and growth, and the social situation in Jamaica, which was deteriorating as a result of tremendous political upheaval. In addition, I had to think of Sylvan's own professional development. Eventually I went to see the university's vice chancellor, Sir Roy Marshall, another Barbadian, who in his droll manner said, "But, Champ, you cannot leave, you know." Another one of my English colleagues encouraged me to accept the offer in Britain and gave as his reason the fact that he would be absolutely tickled to see a black Barbadian telling white Englishmen what to eat. Eventually Sylvan and I agreed that I should stay, and on 11 April 1972, I wrote to the Medical Research Council as follows: "It is with some regret that I must ask that I be not considered any further for the directorship of the Dunn laboratory. After having seen it, I was very enthusiastic about the role it could play in both basic and applied nutrition on a national and international scale. This made my decision even more difficult, but after returning home and considering also the work that must be done here, I thought it best to concentrate my efforts locally."

I wrote to Professor Rosenheim to tell him of my decision and my appointment, and he replied as follows:

> Dear Professor,
> I was thrilled to get your letter and to hear of your decision and your appointment. I am delighted and send you my very warmest congratulations and the best of good wishes. I'm sure that you will do a wonderful job and that the Caribbean will benefit from your decision and that you will never regret it. I have felt a little guilty after our discussion that I had perhaps given you advice although I said I would not. I am sure that I left you in no doubt as to what I thought you should do and I am terribly pleased.

And he ended with this comment in his own handwriting: "Well done, Champ!"

I was formerly appointed professor of medicine as of 1 June 1972, and indeed my academic rise had been nothing short of meteoric, from registrar in medicine in 1962 to professor of medicine in 1972. I received numerous cards, telegrams and letters of congratulation, including an amusing one from Sir Harold Himsworth. He offered me what he considered a critical piece of advice, which was to avoid meetings which were a waste of time if they did not contribute to clinical work or, more importantly, my research.

THE DEPARTMENT OF MEDICINE

The first few months as professor were challenging, as not having been involved in direct patient care for seven years, I had to devote considerable time to bringing myself up to speed. This meant a prodigious amount of reading and long hours spent with patients, but in the fullness of time, I regained my clinical skills and was able to indulge my innate love of teaching, especially physical diagnosis. It is one of the great pleasures of academia to be able to transmit an idea to young people and to see them grasp and internalize it. I still meet men and women in the Caribbean and beyond who recall with pleasure being taught by me. Eventually I became head of the department in 1976 after a mild internal conflict. There had been a tacit agreement on my appointment that the headship of the department would rotate to me after three years, and it had not.

One of the first issues which struck me on entering the department was the manner in which we trained our successors, as reflected in our system of postgraduate training and examination. The need for postgraduate training had long been recognized by the ministers of health and the Faculty of Medicine. The presence of the SS *Hope* in Kingston in 1970 contributed to a resurgence of the idea that the time had come for a formal programme of postgraduate training. The dean of the Faculty of Medicine, Dr Mohan Ragbeer, approached the Hope Foundation with a suggestion that it participate in initiating and continuing a postgraduate training programme in a few select disciplines. It was felt that if training were available locally, fewer physicians would seek training in the United States, the United Kingdom or Canada, as this early postgraduate exposure abroad contributed significantly to the brain drain.[1]

The programme would start in Jamaica and be expanded to other West Indian islands in due course. Eventually, in 1971, the University of the West Indies, the Government of Jamaica and the Hope Foundation signed a memorandum of understanding to establish programmes in postgraduate medical education in Jamaica in a few select specialties.[2] The memorandum noted specifically the attraction of postgraduate training in North America because of its structured nature. In view of the problem of staff shortage, the Hope Foundation agreed to provide staff tutors and senior residents in various disciplines – initially paediatrics, surgery and general medicine, with obstetrics and gynaecology and pathology developed later. The university accepted responsibility for developing the programme as well as for academic control and supervision, which included evaluation, examination and the award of postgraduate degrees and diplomas. It was decided that the university would be the certifying body for the specialist qualification, which would be a doctorate in medicine (DM). The specialists in all disciplines graduated with a DM but qualified their specialty, for example, DM (Surgery).

The programme started slowly and with some difficulty over the number of training positions available, as the existing junior service posts essentially became the training positions. Considerable credit must be given to the Government of Jamaica for extending itself to make additional positions available at the University Hospital of the West Indies for training purposes. The personnel supplied under the aegis of the Hope Foundation were excellent, and the personal characteristics of the senior administrative staff – Rufus Morrow and Richard Meltzer – contributed significantly to the eventual success of the programme. Support to the Department of Medicine was provided not only in the shape of general internists but also through a successful rotational scheme with the University of Toronto, which had neurologists rotating for various periods through the department.

I was the first person from outside the United Kingdom to be invited to be an examiner in the MRCP examination in London, and this gave me a keen appreciation of the nature of postgraduate examinations and exposed the limitations of using an examination as the sole seal of proficiency in medicine. I compared it with my exposure to the residency approach with increasing responsibility that characterizes the American system. I was also fortunate to be invited to participate in the examination for the Fellowship of the Royal College of Physicians and Surgeons of Canada, which approximated better the Internal Medicine Boards of the United States. I should note, however, that the climate in Britain had changed or was changing to have the MRCP exam as the gateway to further and more structured training rather than as a certificate of proficiency in internal medicine. It was clear to me that the international trend was towards an apprentice-type system with graded responsibility. It is a pleasure now to see most of the physicians in the Caribbean as graduates of our training programme, including the former vice chancellor of the University of the West Indies.

The start was not without its problems. One of them was to ensure that our examinations and examiners focused on the fitness of the students to be physicians and deal with real problems. One of the early candidates who had not gone through the structured programme came to the final examination and was quizzed on what I thought were irrelevant facts. At the examiners' final meeting, it was decided to fail him, and for the first time and in a public meeting, I wept openly. The student had been an honours graduate in his undergraduate examination, and I felt the decision to fail him was unfair. I swore that it would never happen again, and I introduced structured teaching sessions for the trainees and was firm with examiners as to the kind of questions to be put. I would not have questions that were merely an exercise in memory culture. I introduced multiple-choice questions and was fortunate to obtain a bank of several thousand questions from a Canadian source which could be adapted for our use. When I was questioned by colleagues accustomed only to essay-type questions, I would reply that I would be happy if a candidate knew the answer to every one of the multiple-choice questions in the bank.

I had not been long in the department when I was invited to the opening of a new nutrition research centre in Chiang Mai, Thailand, to speak on mineral metabolism in protein calorie malnutrition. I was flattered, as the participants included some of the most respected and distinguished investigators in the field. The conference went well, and I recall that the centre was opened by the king of Thailand himself in a grand ceremony. On my flight from Chiang Mai to Bangkok, I sat beside Carl Taylor, a professor from Johns Hopkins School of Public Health. We discussed our respective work, and I recall with amazement and some amusement his asking me why I did not do something useful with my life and work in public health. This was now the second time I had been challenged in this manner.

The desirability of linkages with African universities had been mooted for some time, and the idea was strengthened by Dr Oluwasanmi, vice chancellor of the University of Ife, when he gave the graduation address at our university in 1971. The proposal also found favour with our vice chancellor, Sir Roy Marshall, who had spent two years in the University of Ife as dean of law.

The Commonwealth Foundation supported a visit of seven of us to universities in Nigeria, Ghana and Sierra Leone.[3] The team was led by Professor Leslie Robinson, pro-vice-chancellor (planning), and included colleagues from economics, history, engineering, agriculture and chemistry in the University of Guyana. I visited six universities in Nigeria, one in Ghana and one in Sierra Leone. The main discussions were around curriculum development, teaching, student and faculty exchange and research projects of mutual interest. We were struck by the similarities between

The Professor of Medicine: My Appointment

our university and the University of Ibadan, as both had been founded at the same time as part of the thrust towards tertiary education in the colonies.

It was interesting to compare clinical medicine in Nigeria with practice in Jamaica, considering that we shared ethnic backgrounds. The presence, for example, of some aspects of cardiovascular disease such as hypertension and strokes and the manifestations of diabetes strengthened my conviction about the uselessness of the term "tropical medicine". There were, however, some unexplained particularities in that some conditions such as systemic lupus erythematosus, which was common in Jamaica, was exceedingly rare in Nigeria. It was refreshing to see the insistence on clinical skills, which we too emphasized so much in our teaching.

One of the most memorable parts of the trip was a visit to El Mina and Cape Coast castles in Ghana. In Cape Coast we went into the holding cell, saw the stanchions to which the slaves were bolted, and looked down to the sea where the long boats had waited to be loaded with the slaves as they passed through "the gate of no return". There was not a dry eye in the group, as we could picture the misery below, while the traffickers would have been singing and partying above. This brought home more than any book or film the reality of the slave trade and the historical ties that bound so many of us to Africa.

There was enthusiasm for several proposals for visits and exchanges, but perhaps one of the major benefits was that the academics could get to know one another. A concrete result was the exchange of examiners in medicine and surgery, and I examined twice in Ibadan at their final medical examinations and entertained several of their professors in our examinations. It was also recommended that the governments of the two regions which operated airlines should consider the possibility of an air service link between the West Indies and West Africa, but this never materialized.

The visit was a learning experience for other reasons. I was supposed to join the team after my visit to Thailand. I flew from Bangkok to Rome to take Nigeria Airways to Lagos, but on arrival at the airport in Rome, I was told blithely by the Nigeria Airways representative that the flight had been cancelled a week before. I was both astounded and annoyed but was comforted somewhat by a kind Alitalia pilot who took me back to my hotel in his red Ferrari. I duly took the Alitalia flight the next day to Lagos and got a lesson in corruption that I will never forget.

When I landed and went to Immigration, a young man approached and asked for my passport so that he could help me. I indicated to him that I needed no help, because I spoke English. As a result, I was made to wait until every other passenger had been cleared before the immigration officer even spoke to me. Having now learned my lesson, when the skycap took my luggage to the domestic terminal en route to Ibadan and told me that the flight was overbooked but if I treated him well he could speak with the agent and get me a seat, I agreed instantly and paid him handsomely. To my chagrin, when I did board the flight to Ibadan, the plane was half empty.

In 1977, I was awarded the prestigious Sir Arthur Sims Commonwealth Travelling Professorship by the Royal College of Physicians and Surgeons. The professor was required to visit the United Kingdom and other Commonwealth countries, and one of the stipulations was that he be accompanied by his wife. It would involve lectures, seminars, clinical teaching and a round of social activities. Sylvan and I elected to visit England, Scotland, Ireland and Canada, and the most guarded piece of luggage, which was always hand-carried, was a bag with about two hundred slides which I had made personally. The travelling professorship experience was a rich one in which I both learned and taught my hosts about my university and its programmes.

Caribbean physicians of my day prided themselves on their clinical acumen and diagnostic skills, and I was pleased to be able to demonstrate these on several occasions during this tour. I was presented the dossier of a case at a seminar in Ottawa, Canada, and was told that several visiting physicians had been given the same case and failed to make the correct diagnosis. I recall the applause which attended my analysis and final diagnosis that the patient had died from drinking methyl alcohol.

There was one poignant moment in Montreal, when I was accompanying the senior physician on his ward round, and we came to a patient who had presented with paralysis of his legs because multiple myeloma had invaded his spine. The patient related how he had visited several doctors complaining of back pain, and the diagnosis had been missed. He wept, saying that

The Professor of Medicine: My Appointment

his cousin Alan was a doctor, and had he been there, this never would have happened to him, as Alan would have made the correct diagnosis. The patient was Barbadian, and when I questioned him about the village from which he came and his relatives, we appreciated that I was in fact the cousin to whom he was referring. I wept with him.

These were turbulent political times in Jamaica. The charismatic Michael Manley was prime minister and had enthused the population with his version of democratic socialism. This found echo on the university campus, and there was considerable fervour for democratic governance of the university in which all workers from professors to gardeners had equal voice. I asked our departmental maid if she thought it was a good idea for her and the handyman to participate in our departmental meetings. She was amused at the suggestion and politely but emphatically declined.

There were several strikes on campus during examination time, and in one of them, one of our lecturers, Dr Cecil Mac Iver, apparently breached the barricade en route to our clinical-pathology conference, which was being held with the participation of our external examiners. In the middle of the conference, a crowd of workers burst in, led by Dr Trevor Munroe, a lecturer in government and head of the workers' union. They approached Dr Mac Iver menacingly, accused him of hitting one of the strikers at the barricade, and announced loudly that they were there to make a citizens' arrest. There was bedlam, with the academic staff and myself standing around Dr Mac Iver. Eventually good sense prevailed, the invading crowd retired, and we proceeded with our conference. One external examiner subsequently commented that it was one of the more interesting academic experiences he had ever had.

During this period, there was apparently a rumour that the professor of surgery and I were to be attacked as a mechanism of destabilizing the campus. Apparently one of my colleagues alerted the minister of home affairs, Dudley Thompson, about this, and on the night of the supposed attack, there was a helicopter circling my house and shining its light all around it. When Sylvan enquired about this unusual attention, I dismissed it and said she was not to worry. The next morning, however, when I was at work, she received a call from the minister enquiring whether the night had passed uneventfully. She was naturally nonplussed about this, but when the vice chancellor, Aston Preston, phoned later to find out if I was safe, she became incensed and telephoned me in anger to find out why I had not told her all about this. It took a long time for her to forgive me. One of the consequences was that for many nights there were armed soldiers on my street and an armed guard on my veranda. But deciding this was not a good image for my young children, I suggested that he be removed. I would take my chances. I was adamant that these threats should not disturb my routine, and during the nights when my clinical service was receiving patients, I would routinely leave home at all hours to see them in hospital.

The department faced some fundamental challenges. When the university began, and there was clinical teaching in the hospital, all physicians practised primarily as generalists, and any additional expertise did not require separate facilities. Patients with cardiac problems were admitted to the general wards; gastroenterology was rudimentary. But with the advances in medicine, both in terms of basic knowledge and the technology available, there was inevitable pressure to have individual specialty facilities: neurology, haematology, nephrology and so on. This tension was never quite resolved during my time as professor of medicine. Exposure to clinical sub-specialization led to the belief that while the individual patient might benefit from special expertise, there was the danger that the medical student might not grasp the fundamentals of general medicine upon which specialty expertise would be grafted. It has been interesting and salutary to see one of our own graduates, Herbert Ho Ping Kong, make a tremendous reputation for himself as a specialist in general internal medicine in Toronto. He has become deservedly famous as the person to whom patients with difficult problems are referred, as he is able to bring to bear a breadth of general clinical knowledge and experience.[4]

Small clinical departments, such as the department was at that time, will always face as the norm the challenge of having its staff see patients in the departments or at least in the hospital. There will be the tendency to compare with physicians of similar vintage and experience in private practice who earn considerably more. This has never been solved satisfactorily anywhere. Academic physicians who are not readily available to consult with their juniors and oversee their patients have great difficulty discharging their basic academic responsibilities. The creation of practice facilities

The Professor of Medicine: My Appointment

within or in close proximity to the academic unit may provide a partial answer, and this was one of the reasons for the construction of an annex to the Department of Medicine which would provide additional space and facilitate increased geographical clinical practice.

The space constraints in the department were becoming ever more acute. In 1976, when I became head, I approached the vice chancellor about the possibility of an extension to the building. He agreed tentatively but made it clear that we would have to raise the necessary funding ourselves. I spoke to Professor Hugh Wynter, head of the Department of Obstetrics and Gynaecology, and he agreed that this would be a joint project, as his department, which occupied the floor below ours, also required space. Not daunted, we formed a building committee and began with a naive idea that our requests would only target former patients. Eventually we launched an appeal for J$300,000, and many of our patients did respond but with small contributions. There cannot have been any professional association, embassy, business person who did not receive a request for support. Letters were sent to the most unlikely persons, for example to Muhammad Ali, who had just lost his heavyweight crown on the pretext that he was a "champ", as was I. The cost of the building eventually increased to J$478,000, but we raised approximately J$350,000, and the university assisted with the remainder. We were fortunate to have Jim Lim, who was then managing director of Desnoes and Geddes, a major Jamaican firm, as chair of our committee, and he was ably assisted by his wife, Bea. My friend Leonard Berkeley made a pro bono contribution of the services of his quantity surveyor firm, and Joan Parnell was a most efficient project coordinator. The largest contributor of US$50,000 came from the Alcoa Foundation. The building was formally opened in January 1981.

It was not easy to stimulate research in the department. My own research team continued to do well and was considered one of the best in the world. It was well supported financially and attracted West Indian and foreign fellows. We concentrated mainly on intermediary metabolism and the problems of renal biochemistry, including the mechanism by which the kidney made glucose while producing ammonia in response to an acid load. I am still amazed at the work done in a small laboratory in the Department of Medicine with corridor space annexed for installation of some of the major equipment. I collaborated with colleagues in other departments in research on several aspects of clinical nephrology and supervised several master's and doctoral students. But for the rest of the staff, with a few exceptions there were no defined teams or schools of inquiry, and the senior staff really did not make research a priority, instead concentrating on teaching. Nevertheless, some of the staff pursued individual research efforts leading to doctoral dissertations.

The management of the department represented some difficulties for several reasons. First it is always difficult to create a team out of highly qualified specialists, confident of their own expertise, self-sufficient and not convinced of the need for collective action. In addition, I was not much older than most of the staff, and that may have led sometimes to issues, but eventually, with equanimity that was often strained and the obvious concentration on the team, I believe I earned their respect and loyalty.

While they were all good colleagues, I must make special mention of Owen Morgan, who is one of nature's gentlemen. He was a first-class neurologist and honest to the core. He is one person whose word is truly his bond. We would have arguments about various aspects of the work, but never was there rancour, and once there was an agreement, I could depend on his loyal support. There was no aspect of managing the department in which he did not participate. I owe him a great debt.

The efficiency of our department was helped enormously by outstanding secretarial support, and I will always be indebted to Noelle Lalor, the senior secretary, for her competence and loyalty. Clinical teaching had been decentralized to Trinidad and Tobago and Barbados, with much of it being done by government physicians in addition to the small university academic staff. We had to be certain that students received the same level of teaching in all three places, but the evidence from examinations showed that they were well taught outside of Mona as well. It is a pleasure to acknowledge the loyalty and support of the academic staff in Trinidad and Tobago and Barbados. It was always a stimulating and enjoyable experience to conduct the final examinations in those countries.

CHAPTER 6

The Beginning of the International Odyssey
Leaving Jamaica

And then in 1981, it became obvious to me that I should leave. Our family by that time was five. We had adopted a baby girl, Carol, in 1965; Andrew was born in 1968 and Adrian in 1970. Sylvan was a lecturer in social work in the university. We now owned a house, and in spite of the problems of living in Jamaica, by and large we were doing well.

It is interesting to reflect on why I left when I did. I go back to one of the bits of advice Professor Rosenheim gave me, although he claimed that he never gave advice – he only helped people to think through their options. But he did "advise" me never to make long-term plans in terms of my career. One should do one's current job to the best of one's ability, and one day there would be an epiphany; it would become clear that it was time to move, and, surprisingly, options would appear.

So in 1981, I was contemplating leaving the university. The department was well staffed, and some of the graduates from our own postgraduate programmes were on staff. The postgraduate programme was well structured – there was a new building, which eased the space constraints, and there were no immediate funding problems. There was harmony with the clinical teaching units in Trinidad and Tobago and Barbados with clear recognition of the authority of the chair of the department. Perhaps it was also becoming clearer to me that it was increasingly difficult, if not impossible, to work at the laboratory bench which I enjoyed. I could supervise research, find funding for it and ensure that the work was published, but the clinical and administrative responsibilities made it difficult to work at the bench for sustained periods.

I had had the good fortune during my periods of study leave to work on my research in several biochemical laboratories. In 1970, I went to Professor Philip Randle's laboratory in the University of Bristol where I worked with two excellent colleagues, Chris Pogson and Ian Longshaw on renal metabolism. I did the same in 1974, when I went to the University of Canterbury, where Chris Pogson had moved. In 1978, I went to the biochemistry department of the University of Granada, Spain. The work was intense and fascinating, as here we had rats swim in a small tank to create the metabolic acidosis that we wished to study. One of the benefits was that my family and I were exposed to the Spanish language and culture. In addition, we were able to visit on several occasions the fabled Alhambra Castle, one of the finest examples of Moorish architecture in southern Spain. One of the Spanish biochemists, Paloma Hortelano, subsequently came to join my laboratory in Jamaica for six months. These enjoyable sojourns in which I could dedicate myself fully to research just emphasized the difficulty in combining it with the responsibilities inherent in being a department chair.

When I announced formally that I was leaving, a symposium was arranged in my honour by Owen Morgan in June 1981, at which I gave a farewell address entitled "Apologia of a Gusanito". An *apologia*, as in the apologia of Socrates, is a speech in defence of something or someone, and a *gusanito* was a little worm, referencing the word that Fidel Castro used for Cubans who fled Cuba for the United States. He called them *gusanos*.

> I would like to speak a little more about our University and its functions. Many of the problems that we encounter, many of the brickbats stem from differences people have – their perception of the image of a University as compared with other corporate organizations. One of my gurus, Alfred P. Sloan is alleged to have said that "the first thing a company needs to do is know its public and know its product". The Ford company knows its business is making motorcars. Ford sets out to find what the customer wants and makes motorcars to suit. Now you ask what is the university's business. Primacy goes to knowledge production and knowledge transmission. The

The Beginning of the International Odyssey: Leaving Jamaica

> Ford Motor Company can determine whether it is successful or not by the number of cars it makes and the amount of profit it makes – a University cannot do that. Many from the outside, many of our political masters do not quite appreciate that the short-term evidence of gain and the evidence of achievement of short-term goals cannot be the only criteria of success in an institution like the University which is committed to knowledge production and knowledge transmission. Our University is still young and we sell it short if we encourage our Masters and encourage our critics to judge us by the short-term realization of the kinds of goals which Ford and General Motors have.

I left some charges. The first was that this institution must be irrevocably committed to research. I did not hide my view that if we allowed to prevail the doctrine that research is a luxury, that there is any discipline in which research is not proper and necessary, then we would not be true to the principles of academia.

I expanded on the research theme:

> Elsewhere I have referred to the steps through which research has gone in the University. Our founding fathers were basically phenomenologists and it is remarkable how quickly we built up a reputation for good research. We must be careful that good clinical observation is not being passed over as trivial and we must frown upon the tendency to say that all has been discovered. In fact, it has not. We in the University are in a better position than our counterparts in most universities of the world. We have many of the medical problems of the developing world and some of those of the developed world, and even though some of you may not believe it, technologically we are probably decades ahead of most medical schools of our size in the developing world. There are new numerous genuine clinical problems here to engage us at the level of clinical observation and also at the level of basic investigation relevant to clinical problems.

The final charge was as follows:

> The last thing I would ask you to do is to avoid arrogance of materialistic medicine. I have been rereading recently Bronowski's The Ascent of Man and he describes graphically how Galileo met his fate, because he dared to bring into argument the relationship between things scientific and things

spiritual. The counterpart to Galileo is Descartes who attempted to separate matter and soul, perhaps as a device to disengage biology from the church. A psychiatrist from Harvard, Leon Eisenberg analyses the Cartesian approach to science and shows how Descartes as a devout Catholic had great difficulty with his own view of physiology. But as Eisenberg points out, this Cartesian dichotomy has now gone too far and we have become too attuned to the physical aspect of patient care. The momentum of technological imperative to do what we have the virtuosity to do often brings the physician into conflict with what the patient seeks from him or her. The patient has an illness and in many cases the physician has a tendency to see and treat disease only as a malady of structure and function. As physicians we are not often as conscious as we should be of the individual's role in the social system.

I ended by saying the following:

I have no fear about the future of this institution because of the obvious quality of our graduates. One of my favourite poets, A.E. Houseman, who in describing Queen Victoria's Jubilee was explaining why there was nothing to fear about England's future. He said:
God will save her, fear ye not
be you the men you have been
get you the sons your fathers got
and God will save the Queen.
I am convinced that many of us have gotten the kind of academic sons who will beget the sons who will ensure the future of our institution.

And so I left Jamaica in August 1981 for Washington, DC, to join the Pan American Health Organization.

THE PAN AMERICAN HEALTH ORGANIZATION

In 1970, John Waterlow asked me to be a member of the PAHO Advisory Committee on Medical Research, of which he was chairman. This committee comprised distinguished scientists from the Americas and, over the course of my association with it, included several Nobel Prize winners – Sune Bergstrom, Luis Leloir, Cesar Milstein, Fred Robbins, Tom Weller.

The Beginning of the International Odyssey: Leaving Jamaica

We looked at various regional health problems and advised the director on possible research opportunities. As I wrote English reasonably well, I was asked to be rapporteur and to prepare the final report. At the first meeting I prepared my report, only to have it edited heavily by Magaly Galdo, who was then secretary in the Office of Research Coordination. To say I was upset is to put it mildly, but she was correct, and thereafter I took much more care over my reports. Eventually I became chair of the committee and was often critical of the response by the organization to our recommendations. In 1980, Dr Perez-Miravete, head of the Office of Research Coordination, retired, and the director, Dr Hector Acuna, offered me the position at the level of P6.

This offer came at a critical time in my career, as I was also offered a position at the same level in the World Health Organization (WHO) in Geneva in the Tropical Disease Research Programme. This brought into relief the sage advice I had received from Professor Rosenheim, that I should never worry about my career. I should concentrate on the job in hand, and the next opportunity would come as an epiphany. This was such a moment as he had described: the options were before me, and I had to decide whether to leave the university.

Eventually, after much discussion and consultation in the family, we decided to go to Washington for a year in the first instance, so I took a sabbatical year. I chose the Pan American Health Organization partly because of my previous experience with that area of work and the possibility of painting on a larger canvas, and also because I felt it would permit me to stay in touch with the Caribbean. Leaving was emotional, and our vice chancellor, Aston Preston, was among many people from within and without the university who were reluctant to see me go but still wished me good luck.

The Pan American Health Organization was established in 1902 and is the world's oldest international health organization.[1] It had its genesis in concern for the spread of infectious diseases, which were a barrier to trade and commerce. Thus, towards the end of the nineteenth century, several global sanitary conferences tried to adopt some common approach to the problem. The end of that century also saw movement towards cooperation among the republics of the Americas, and in 1890 the precursor of the current Organization of American States was formed as the International Union of American States. In its second conference in Mexico in 1902, the States mandated a meeting of representatives of their health organizations to discuss matters of mutual interest and to create a bureau to formulate uniform sanitary laws and regulations. The meeting was held in Washington in December 1902, in the Willard Hotel, which still exists in the same location, and concentrated on the regional threat of infectious diseases. That meeting was also significant in that Carlos Finlay from Cuba proposed that a mosquito was the vector of the agent carrying yellow fever. The other significant development was the decision to establish a central sanitary bureau with permanent headquarters in Washington, DC, for the purpose of rendering effective service to the different republics. The bureau's basic role was to be the repository of and disseminator of information, particularly in reference to infectious diseases, mainly cholera and yellow fever. At the seventh conference in Havana, Cuba, in 1924, a Pan American Sanitary Code was drafted and ratified and still remains the treaty basis that sustains PAHO's operations. Over the years, the bureau's activities predominantly in information sharing increased in large part due to the initiative of Dr Hugh Cummings, who was director from 1920 to 1947 as well as being surgeon-general of the United States.

The first crisis in the bureau's existence came with the formation of the World Health Organization in 1948. A major point of discussion was the relationship between the new global organization and the bureau, which was by then the oldest and most important intergovernmental health agency in the world. One view was that the regional organization should be incorporated fully into WHO. But the delegates from the Americas stoutly defended their organization, and eventually the compromise was reached in an agreement that said that "the regional organization shall in due course be integrated with the organization (WHO). This integration shall be effected as soon as practicable through common action based on mutual consent of the competent authorities expressed through the organizations concerned."

"Due course" has not arrived, and there has been no substantive attempt to arrive at "mutual consent". It was agreed that the bureau would serve as the regional office of WHO in the Americas. Staff which hitherto had been detailed from the United States Public Health Service was withdrawn, and the bureau, now renamed the Pan American Sanitary Organization, began to hire international staff. The independence of the regional organization was facilitated by the fact that its budget, thanks to the efforts of its director, Dr Fred Soper, was larger than that of the WHO.[2] In 1958, the name was changed from the Pan American Sanitary Organization to the Pan American Health Organization, which as currently understood represents the Pan American Sanitary Bureau, or Secretariat, plus its member states. It has grown to encompass all the independent countries of the Americas, Great Britain, France and the Kingdom of the Netherlands, representing their dependencies in the region. PAHO is headquartered in Washington, DC, and has representative offices in virtually every country in the Americas. It is headed by a director who also serves as the regional director for the WHO in the Americas.

The organization has undergone several administrative changes, but its essential function remains the same – to be a leader in assisting the countries of the Americas in the quest for better health for all their peoples. It is supported by quota contributions from member countries, plus a contribution from the World Health Organization in view of its role as the regional office of WHO in the Americas. Its directors were US citizens until 1958, when Dr Abraham Horwitz from Chile became director and served until 1975. He was succeeded by Dr Hector Acuna from Mexico, 1975 to 1983, and then Dr Carlyle Guerra de Macedo from Brazil, 1983 to 1995. When I assumed the directorship, the international staff spread all over the Americas was over a thousand and was supplemented by a larger number of staff hired locally. The projected budget for the biennium 1996 to 1998 was approximately a quarter of US$1 billion.

I was fortunate that there was an excellent group of professionals in the Research Coordination Unit of which I was head, and the most outstanding of them was Gabriel Schmunis, an Argentinian infectious disease specialist. In spite of the fact that he had aspired to the position of head of the unit, he was the essence of loyalty and support, and he and his wife have continued to be among our closest friends. The adaptation was not without its difficulties. First, there was the problem of putting into practice my idea of having a unitary focus for a unit in which individuals were carrying on with their own individual interests. I had to adjust to the need for various clearances of correspondence. Coming as I did from being head of a department, it was sometimes difficult to accept that because the unit was within the Division of Human Resources, memoranda had to be cleared by the administrator and then the division chief. To be fair, they were both excellent and in retrospect remarkably tolerant. The division chief, José Roberto Ferreira, a Brazilian, was exceptionally kind and generous, and even before I assumed duty, he took me to lunch and predicted that one day I would become director of the organization. He foresaw the Caribbean countries assuming more and more influence in PAHO, and as the senior Caribbean person in the organization, I would have an excellent chance of being director at some time in the future.

The language was another problem, but after a couple weeks of a tutor who told me that the best thing was to be bold, to "Go ahead and murder the language", I took her advice. Some of the results were hilarious and occasionally embarrassing, but I progressed satisfactorily, because of my background in Latin, and a certain facility with language, as well as not being inhibited by my mistakes. One day I saw our administrator wearing a beautiful shell necklace and gallantly said to her in perfect Castilian Spanish, "Que linda es su concha." She blushed, stammered and suggested that I repeat that to one of my Spanish-speaking colleagues, which I did. He explained to me that the word *concha* was the vernacular in Latin America for vagina, and I had complimented her on its beauty.

It took considerable patience to get accustomed to the style of management predominant in the organization. I found that decision-making was slow and, to my taste, not optimally efficient. The need for what seemed minor decisions to be taken at higher levels often amazed me. One example stands out in my mind. I arranged a meeting of the PAHO Advisory Committee on Medical Research for which our unit provided the secretariat, and the director, Dr Acuna himself, wished to see how the seating at the head table was to be arranged. Even the colour of the covers of some reports had to be vetted at that level.

The Beginning of the International Odyssey: Leaving Jamaica

POLITICS IN PAHO

The forthcoming election of the new director was the topic of intense discussion at the time I joined. There were two main candidates for the directorship, which would be decided in 1982 at the meeting of the PAHO Sanitary Conference. One was Dr David Tejada, a Peruvian who was then assistant director general of WHO in Geneva, and the other was Dr Carlyle Guerra de Macedo, a relatively unknown Brazilian. The United States openly supported Tejada, allegedly because Dr Macedo's politics were very much to the left. I was then still naive and had thought that elections were a matter for the politicians. I could not quite understand why staff members were so involved. I was a bit perplexed when Jose Teruel, a fellow Brazilian, brought Dr Macedo to see me, because he thought I had influence in the Caribbean. Dr Macedo was elected in 1982 with strong support from the Caribbean countries, and that influenced my future status in PAHO considerably.

Dr Macedo had made a commitment to the CARICOM countries that a Caribbean national would have a prominent position in his administration. That obviously was one of the ways through which he achieved their support. After being elected, he restructured the secretariat to have two main technical divisions and promised that someone from the Caribbean would head one of these. Again in my naivety I thought he would select the person he felt to be the most competent, and I knew I was being considered, but I did nothing, expecting to be evaluated on my merit.

Then one day Dr Macedo called me to his office and told me that he had consulted the Caribbean governments. He showed me the list of responses. Some of them had supported me and others were supporting Harold Drayton, who was then a PAHO staff member in Human Resources Development in the PAHO office in Barbados. I knew Harry Drayton, knew that he was very competent, had done a good job in Barbados and was well thought of by Dr Philip Boyd, who was then head of the CARICOM health desk. I quickly found out that supported by friends within PAHO, he had been actively lobbying the Caribbean governments for the position. I contacted the Barbados, Jamaican and Bahamas governments and informed them of the Drayton lobby. My conversation with the minister of health of Barbados, Don Blackman, was colourful, and he remarked in cryptic fashion,

"They are playing some very dirty pool." Harry's ingenious argument was that I was already at a high level in PAHO, and the Caribbean would be better off having another person, himself, at a high level there.

Suffice it to say that there was rapid action by Barbados and Jamaica especially, and the permanent secretary of health of the Bahamas, Hal Munnings, immediately phoned and wrote to Dr Macedo. These three tipped the scale, and he could then announce that he was appointing me as director of health programmes and Luis Carlos Ochoa, a Colombian, as director of health systems. I got to know that there were six votes for me and five for Drayton. I have a copy of a telegram from the minister of health of Guyana expressing enthusiastic support for Drayton. It is interesting that when that minister left office, I was instrumental in furthering his training in public health and having him appointed to a post within PAHO. There were some immediate comical consequences. I had been sharing a car pool with the head of one of the technical departments in my new area, but with the new arrangement, I became his supervisor. He immediately told me that he preferred we carpool no more, and it was more convenient for us to drive to work separately.

DIRECTOR, HEALTH PROGRAMS DEVELOPMENT

The Health Programs Development area was responsible for PAHO's programmes in maternal and child health, communicable and chronic non-communicable diseases, immunization, environmental health and veterinary public health. I had little difficulty understanding the nature of the technical issues involved in my area, but I felt that the main task would be to streamline the management practices. I developed a background paper on the management approach I intended to adopt, with emphasis on clarity of programming of the technical cooperation, which was accepted by Dr Macedo. I knew that with professionals at this level, the better approach was achieving agreement through discussion, dialogue and convincing argument rather than through threats or sanctions, even if that were possible. I was not convinced that there was uniform conceptualization of what constituted our technical cooperation, and there was confusion about the difference between technical assistance and technical cooperation.

The Beginning of the International Odyssey: Leaving Jamaica

During this period, I persuaded Dr Macedo to introduce formal annual evaluations of the organization's work. These began as conversations around the director's conference table at the end of the year and grew to be highly structured affairs, based on a format I developed. Fortunately or unfortunately, his enthusiasm and tolerance for long hours contributed to these being marathon sessions dreaded by all the staff. At the end of his directorship, these would last into the small hours of the morning, and amazingly, he would never fade or lose attention even as many around the table were nodding away.

I cannot say that everyone in my area accepted my direction kindly, but this was not new to me. I could sympathize with those who were previously heads of their departments reporting to the director and who were now being supervised by a relative newcomer and a non-Latin to boot. But to their credit, we were able to maintain a professional relationship based on mutual respect, and there were significant advances in the work of the area.

I enjoyed particularly the interaction with the technical units and the discussions of the organization of the programmes, especially at the country level. The programme on immunization was one of the stars of my area, as it was headed by an extraordinarily talented Brazilian epidemiologist, Dr Ciro de Quadros, and it had embarked on an ambitious programme for the eradication of poliomyelitis from the Americas. This programme was remarkably successful, as the Americas was indeed the first region in the world to eradicate poliomyelitis.[3] I have always cited the success as being due to excellent leadership, adequate funding, commitment on the part of all the governments, and observance and implementation of some basic organizational principles.

Over time I rejected several offers to leave PAHO. Dr Halfdan Mahler, the director general of WHO, proposed that I come to Geneva to be head of the Special Programme of Research and Training in Tropical Diseases. When I respectfully declined, he asked if there was anything I wished. To which I replied, simply, money for the programme on acute respiratory infections. He agreed and did indeed allot significant additional funding for this programme. The programme on acute respiratory infections was of special interest to me, as on my joining PAHO it had become obvious that this was a relatively neglected major cause of childhood morbidity and mortality. Gabriel Schmunis and I collaborated with others in PAHO in writing a book on the topic,[4] which I believe helped to stimulate programme interest, and subsequently from my position as head of the area, I could assist in incorporating this into the programme of Integrated Management of Childhood Illness.

In 1987, the assistant director, Ramon Alvarez Gutierrez, retired. He was Mexican and always elegant, with a remarkable appreciation of the problems of administration in an international organization. He never left a file or paper on his desk when he left work for the day, and he rarely stayed late. He advised me to be careful of what he described as the "Jell-O principle", which he said applied to some staff. One would give a clear instruction, or tap the Jell-O, there would be lateral movement, and soon it would become clear that nothing had changed: the Jell-O had settled back to its original level surface. He had a keen sense of the politically possible and where decisions should be taken.

On his departure, Luis Carlos Ochoa was appointed assistant director. I was a bit chagrined but somewhat mollified when Dr Macedo explained to me the pressure he had from the Latin countries to have a Latin in that position. Luis Carlos retired in 1990, and that is when I was appointed assistant director.

ASSISTANT DIRECTOR

The main responsibility was supervision of the country offices and the technical cooperation with countries. The assistant director was supported by four country analysts, who were responsible for various groupings of the countries. There was a succession of highly competent Caribbean women responsible for the CARICOM countries – Dorothy Blake, Karen Sealey, Lilian Reneau and Kathleen Israel. I also had responsibility for supervising the programmes on Women, Health and Development and that of Disaster Preparedness. There were numerous mini crises, such as maintaining the cooperation with Haiti after the overthrow of President Aristide and the rule by a military government. PAHO found itself buying petroleum from Venezuela and transporting it to Haiti to be distributed to the

The Beginning of the International Odyssey: Leaving Jamaica

non-governmental organizations responsible for much of the health of the Haitian people. The PAHO representative in Haiti at that time, Dr Marie-Andre Diouf, who was originally from Senegal, did a remarkable job in keeping PAHO out of the political line of fire and still supporting health work there.

I visited every one of the PAHO country offices and became more familiar with the challenges of technical cooperation to governments that differed widely in technical expertise and financial resources. I developed an even greater degree of appreciation of the central and critical role these offices played in positioning PAHO as the key player in regional health affairs.

In 1990, Dr Macedo elected to run for a third term, and there was scepticism about this among some of the larger countries. The Canadian representative, Norbert Prefontaine, came to my office and asked whether I would run against him, as Canada was not enthusiastic about his having a third term. I declined and said I would do everything to support his reelection. However, just before leaving, he said that I should consider being director when he demitted office in 1994. I did indeed lobby the Caribbean governments to support Dr Macedo en bloc, and eventually he was elected unopposed.

In 1990, however, Dr Macedo also decided to run for the directorship of WHO, and I was amazed to learn, not from him, that he had proposed to Dr Guillermo Soberon, then minister of health of Mexico, that he become director of PAHO. Apparently he pointed out to Soberon that he would need my support and that of the Caribbean countries, and should I decide to run when he left, Soberon's election would be doubtful, as there was already a suggestion of a non-Latin becoming director. I was intrigued when Dr Soberon, whom I had known and respected as an eminent public health leader and who had been a member of the PAHO Advisory Committee on Medical Research while I was a member in the 1970s, approached me and asked my intentions. He was frank about his discussions and plans. By then I was less politically naive and made the proper noises about collaboration but indicated that I would have to discuss this with my government. The problem never arose, as Dr Macedo was defeated by the Japanese Hiroshi Nakajima.

ENGAGEMENT WITH THE CARIBBEAN

I perceived from the start that there was an uneasy relationship between PAHO and the Caribbean countries. These countries, recently independent, had come late and a bit timidly to the inter-American system. It was noticeable that the Caribbean countries were regarded as somewhat of a problem by some of the senior management of PAHO, and on the other hand, there was scepticism in the Caribbean about the sufficiency and value of PAHO's resources applied to the region. Part of the problem derived from language. The Caribbean public health officials with whom PAHO staff dealt spoke little or no Spanish, and few of the PAHO staff were really fluent in English. In addition, there were few Caribbean nationals in PAHO.

In 1951, PAHO had divided the region of the Americas into zones for administrative purposes, and the Caribbean countries were managed from the zone office in Caracas, Venezuela. In 1978, an Office of Caribbean Program Coordination was created in Barbados in addition to country offices in Jamaica, Trinidad and Tobago, and Guyana. The concern with the use of PAHO's resources in the Caribbean was not confined to the Caribbean countries, as some of the larger countries questioned whether the organization of the resources was efficient, sometimes with the undertone that too much of the budget was being spent on the small Caribbean countries. Dr Acuna as director was sensitive to any criticism at all, and in meetings of the Caribbean ministers of health, he would address this issue sometimes plaintively. In such a meeting in Belize in 1981, he said:

> PAHO, as a health organization that is administratively and technically geared to serve all member countries of this Western Hemisphere region, has been and is working through its Caribbean Program Coordinator's Office to develop new suggestions to facilitate self-sufficiency in health matters either by strengthening your capabilities or by giving you support through technical cooperation. We seek to establish mechanisms for close collaboration not only within your countries but throughout our hemisphere.
>
> We would like to stress that our structures are not rigid and that we are taking the necessary steps to enhance our technical cooperation in order to contribute more effectively and efficiently to the needs of the emerging nations of the Caribbean and the delivery of health services.

The Beginning of the International Odyssey: Leaving Jamaica

At the meeting of the Directing Council in the same year, however, when he was being questioned sharply, especially by Canada, on PAHO's role in the Caribbean, he announced that he was appointing a task force comprising PAHO staff members to be headed by George Alleyne to examine the use of PAHO's resources in the Caribbean. I had not been consulted, had joined the organization just two months before and clearly had not been apprised of all the background and history of this development.

The terms of reference of the task force were as follows:

1. To analyse current use and distribution of the PAHO financial and human resources in the Caribbean.
2. To analyse the relation of other inputs to the PAHO's programme of technical cooperation in the Caribbean.
3. To analyse the appropriateness of PAHO's current method of giving technical cooperation, especially in the smaller countries.
4. To make recommendations to improve PAHO's programme of technical cooperation in the Caribbean.

The members of the task force were Ken Antrobus, who had been a classmate of mine, Henry Cooney and Miguel Segovia. We visited most of the Caribbean countries, the PAHO offices and centres, and most of the important institutions, and collected a vast amount of data.

In general, the study was regarded as timely and useful by governments and agencies in the Caribbean, and there was an overall positive reaction to the usefulness of PAHO's role in supporting Caribbean health programmes. It was noticeable, however, that the smaller countries were not fully aware of the structure and function of PAHO and did not appreciate the extent of the resources available to them and the way these might be used. There was consensus that overlap and duplication existed in the work of some of the agencies in the Caribbean. This was an issue that merited serious examination and correction.

The health desk of CARICOM was headed by Dr Philip Boyd, one of the icons of public health in the Caribbean and someone who had worked previously in the PAHO zone office in Caracas, Venezuela. He was actually a PAHO staff member who was still being seconded by PAHO to work in

CARICOM and establish its health desk, which indeed under his leadership became the pivot for much cooperation in health in the Caribbean. It was clear to us that he intended to establish a mini PAHO in CARICOM and through the use of grant funding was establishing technical expertise in CARICOM that duplicated that of PAHO. He was a committed Caribbean regionalist, and I believe that this was the motivation for what seemed to the opposition to or reservation about PAHO's technical resources and influence in the area.

There was general agreement by the governments, however, that CARICOM was best suited to formulate, promote and follow up on matters of policy in health. PAHO's technical resources would be better deployed in programme development and support at the country and sub-regional levels. It was clear that coordination among these agencies needed to be strengthened and properly sustained.

This was not the only evaluation of PAHO's work in the Caribbean. The Caribbean Epidemiology Center (CAREC), which was administered by PAHO, was the subject of another evaluation, carried out this time by Carlisle Burton, former permanent secretary in the Ministry of Health in Barbados and a distinguished civil servant who had overseen much of the transformation of the health services there. Philip Boyd argued vigorously for CAREC to pass from PAHO administration to being a CARICOM centre, perhaps the Caribbean equivalent of the Centers for Disease Control and Prevention in the United States.

I was familiar with the history of CAREC. The Rockefeller Foundation had established the Trinidad Virus Research Laboratory under the directorship of Dr Wilbur Downs, a distinguished virologist who had made significant discoveries on virus epidemiology in Trinidad and Tobago. When Downs retired, the centre was transferred to the University of the West Indies, where it functioned as a unit of the university's Department of Microbiology under Leslie Spence, a Trinidadian virologist. It was never a very happy arrangement, and eventually Dr Horwitz offered that PAHO would accept management and direction of the centre, which included appointing its director. The budget would come from PAHO and from quota contributions of the Caribbean governments, with Trinidad and Tobago paying the major share. I was the representative of the University

The Beginning of the International Odyssey: Leaving Jamaica

of the West Indies on the centre's Governing Council for several years and was thus familiar with his history and possibilities.

I had to persuade some of the Caribbean ministers of health and Carlisle Burton himself that the Caribbean was best served by having the centre remain under PAHO's administration. The budget of CAREC would still come from the assessed contributions of the CARICOM member countries and from PAHO. The difficulty in collecting quota payments from the CARICOM countries persuaded me, in spite of my appreciating the need for Caribbean institutions to have Caribbean leadership, that the region was better served by retaining the PAHO administration and the PAHO budget. Subsequent developments with funding for CARICOM entities have justified that position.

Our report to the director made recommendations on some shifts of resources in the region, redesignation of some posts, and we made a strong call for better communication with the Caribbean governments. There was one bold recommendation – "that a study should be made to consider the feasibility of installing a small computer in the CPC's office". It was also clear that there needed to be more cooperation in health in the Caribbean. Given that a new director was elected in 1982, however, scant attention was paid to our conclusions and recommendations at that time, but in time the aspect of cooperation would resurface.

CARIBBEAN COOPERATION

Cooperation in health matters has been an article of faith in the Caribbean for over a century. Georgetown, Demerara, was the site of a British West Indian conference on quarantine in 1888, and no doubt it was the presence and fear of cholera and other infectious diseases which encouraged the search for cooperation. There were periodic West Indian conferences at the beginning of the last century, and the conference of 1921 even recommended a central organization of medical services of the colonies.

It is of interest that little attention was paid to health in the West Indian Federal experiment. Perhaps the view was that health was a matter for the individual states, and in addition, the predominant concern of that era was treating illness, a view that was reinforced by the prominence of illnesses with outward manifestations such as malaria, typhoid fever, cancer, leprosy and so on. The instrumentality of health was not appreciated, and the discipline and practice of public health were in their infancy. There was a West Indian meteorological service, as it was clear that weather affected all countries. There was no Ministry of Health for the federation and only an itinerant medical adviser, who, as far as I know, advised on hospital services and the like and paid little attention to health promotion, disease prevention or population health in general.

It has been argued that the presence of three major institutions led to a resurgence of cooperative action in health after the federation dissolved.[5] These were CARICOM, the University of the West Indies and PAHO/WHO. The 1973 Treaty of Chaguaramas identified health specifically as an area of cooperation. One of the objectives of that treaty was "common services and a cooperation in functional matters such as health, education and culture, communication and industrial relations". But the meetings of the Conference of Health Ministers were designated as one of the institutions of the community, and this institution has been successful in stoking the fires of cooperation in health throughout the region over the years.

The time was ripe for a formal cooperation in health initiative. At the tenth conference of CARICOM ministers responsible for health in 1984 in Dominica, beside the lazy Layou River, Dr Macedo, director of PAHO, who was attending his first meeting of the Caribbean ministers, spelled out in some detail the nature, extent and disposition of PAHO's resources in the region. He outlined the various areas of need and how PAHO could help.

He proposed a new cooperation initiative which was born out of PAHO's experience in the war-torn Central American region of health as a contribution to the Contadora peace process. I helped to prepare his speech, in which he said:

> As I described to you, this new way I have set for the organization to carry out its mission envisages using cooperation in health as a means of building bridges of peace and understanding between peoples. The Caribbean is a sea of tranquility in comparison with some other areas of the Americas. In Central America specifically, tensions, turmoil and open conflict are contributing to an incredible level of soul-destroying hunger, misery and suffering.

The Beginning of the International Odyssey: Leaving Jamaica

PAHO has actively promoted an initiative based on priority health needs to focus international attention and help towards this geographical area. There has been general enthusiasm for this effort, to the extent that the countries of the Contadora group have embraced and supported it. Several agencies have given support and the United Nations Children's Fund (UNICEF) in particular is actively working with us in trying to implement some specific activities.

I am grateful to the countries of the Caribbean which supported this initiative when it was presented to the recent World Health Assembly. I would like to believe that you support the initiative because of your commitment to the idea that all of our destinies are intertwined and health, disease and social deprivation in our neighbors must be a source of concern for us all. We in PAHO are fully conscious of the fact that although your region has been spared the military conflicts of Central America, the impact of the economic crisis and the external debt burden (alluded to in other sections of the conference communiqué) have been no less severe in all your countries.

The policy actions which will flow from structural adjustment for accelerated development and integration approved by Heads of Government are almost certain to have profound implications for health and the entire social sector.

If therefore, this conference were to initiate the formulation of a joint plan of action targeted at the improvement of health conditions in the member states of CARICOM with emphasis on improvement of the health status of vulnerable groups, PAHO would be prepared to collaborate with governments and the Secretariat as we have done in Central America in the identification of priority areas and of relevant national and subregional projects; and to combine resources for implementation over and above those already approved by our Governing Bodies. This would be an initiative for health promotion in the Caribbean basin.

The ministers of health adopted the proposal with alacrity and mandated PAHO and CARICOM to be the secretariat to study and develop it. The initiative, which was named Caribbean Cooperation in Health, was formally launched by the ministers at their annual meeting in Georgetown in June 1986, with subsequent approval by resolution of the XXII PAHO Sanitary Conference in September 1986. I represented PAHO in the joint secretariat and was ably assisted by Dr Halmond Dyer of the Caribbean

Program Coordination and Dr Dorothy Blake, one of the programme analysts in PAHO responsible for the Caribbean. CARICOM was represented by Angela Cropper, its director of functional cooperation. The ultimate goal was to improve the overall health status in the Caribbean, and the Caribbean Cooperation in Health sought to pursue the following specific objectives:

1. To identify and utilize strategic priority areas as entry points for facilitating the more productive use of resources and for promoting TCDC (technical cooperation among developing countries).
2. To develop specific projects as vehicles for improving the whole health delivery system and at the same time impacting on the more critical health sector problems.
3. To improve technical cooperation in health in the Caribbean by stimulating inter-country, inter-agency, and inter-institutional collaboration.
4. To mobilize national and external resources to address the most important problems of the neediest groups and sectors.

Much of the initial focus was on project development with an emphasis on those that promoted cooperation among the countries and the mobilization of external resources. Initially a total of 170 national and regional projects were developed around seven priority areas: environmental protection, including vector control; human resources development; chronic diseases including accidents; strengthening the health systems; food and nutrition; maternal and child health including population issues; and HIV/AIDS. The secretariat was particularly careful about periodic evaluations, which were presented regularly to the Conference of Ministers Responsible for Health. A conclusion from the 1988 evaluation on impact noted the following: "It has not been possible at this early stage to measure the impact of the CCH on the health processes or outcomes in the Caribbean. However, it can be affirmed that the initiative is achieving the objectives which have been established and is having a definitive impact on the way in which the health sector is being viewed and organized in the Caribbean." At the end of 1990, it was estimated that Caribbean Cooperation in Health had succeeded in mobilizing approximately $31 million for national and regional projects.

The Beginning of the International Odyssey: Leaving Jamaica

One of the initiatives for resource mobilization was a ministerial mission to five European capitals in May 1987, which had been preceded by a technical mission in January/February 1987. The ministerial mission comprised Hamilton Green, prime minister of Guyana; Kenneth Baugh, minister of health of Jamaica; Adolphus Freeland, minister of health of Antigua and Barbuda; and Dr Macedo, Dorothy Blake, myself and Angela Cropper. It was successful not only in terms of the financial resources mobilized but also in establishing firmly the health priority needs of the Caribbean region in the countries we visited.

Several anecdotes of the mission will probably not be recorded in official documents. Our visit to Italy was especially noteworthy. All the logistics were finally in order, but on the day before we were to arrive, I received a frantic telephone call from Eduardo Missoni, one of the Italian officials. The prime minister of Guyana's bodyguards wished to enter Italy with their guns, and Immigration would not allow it! The tense impasse was solved by agreeing that the guards would leave their guns in Immigration, and the Italian government would guarantee the security of the prime minister by reserving a whole floor of our hotel for his exclusive use and 24-hour presence of armed guards at the elevator and outside his room. The visit to Italy was successful, with the government committing up to $10 million in support. When Angela Cropper telephoned the CARICOM secretary general to give him the good news, his incredulous reply was "Are you sure it is dollars and not lira?"

We visited the UK Ministry of Overseas Development in London and were received by Baroness Young, minister of state for foreign and commonwealth affairs, and John Caines, permanent secretary in the Ministry of Overseas Development. Mr Caines received us warmly, listened attentively and was effusively congratulatory on the initiative. He was positive about the need for British support to the Caribbean. We left his office with a glow of satisfaction, but after sober reflection, we realized that in fact he had really said nothing and had offered less. One of my colleagues remarked that permanent secretaries do not reach that level in the British civil service without the capacity to say nothing eloquently.

My personal preoccupation with Caribbean health never wavered. Indeed, in an Occasional Paper in 1992 for the West Indian Commission entitled "Whither Caribbean Health", Karen Sealey and I described our major concerns as follows:[6]

- That the current health state of most of the Caribbean people may lead to complacency. There may be diminished attention to the fragility of some of the services and systems which maintain that state and insufficient notice paid to emerging problems.
- That there be greater awareness at all levels of the relationship between health and development. There is a proper focus on economic growth and the indicators of that growth in the region, but it is possible for that focus to take not only centre stage but the wings as well and for policy makers to pay insufficient attention to the importance of health in the development process.
- That there may be lack of clarity as to the determinants of health and well-being and the proper role of the state vis-à-vis other actors in providing or facilitating health care and ensuring that equity of access is preserved.
- That the issues related to women, health and development may be marginalized.
- That health and activities related to health serve to promote and strengthen Caribbean integration.

It is remarkable how so many of those concerns are pertinent even today.

There have been several follow-on programmes of activities bearing the name Caribbean Cooperation in Health, which is now entering its fourth iteration. This cooperation has been successful in the area of infectious diseases, and there has been considerable progress recently on the chronic non-communicable diseases. The region was the first to eliminate poliomyelitis and to mount a successful anti-measles campaign, and the Pan Caribbean Partnership against HIV/AIDS has been lauded as a best practice in HIV prevention and control.

THE CARIBBEAN PUBLIC HEALTH AGENCY

The Caribbean Public Health Agency has been a logical outgrowth of this cooperation in health. In 2010, the director of PAHO, Dr Mirta Roses,

The Beginning of the International Odyssey: Leaving Jamaica

who had worked as an epidemiologist in CAREC, proposed to the secretary general of CARICOM that they should explore the possibility of CAREC passing to Caribbean control. This was in keeping with the philosophy in PAHO that its centres, of which CAREC was one, should pass to national control. The view was that there was enough local talent available to ensure the technical success of national centres, which PAHO would support initially but with gradually decreasing financial contribution. After considerable discussion and technical help, especially from Canada, in 2010 the Caribbean Public Health Agency was born, incorporating CAREC, another PAHO centre, CFNI, in Jamaica, the Caribbean Environmental Health Institute and the Caribbean Drug Testing Laboratory. Thus, after many years, Philip Boyd's vision of a centre in the Caribbean, much like the US Centers for Disease Control and Prevention, would be realized.[7]

CHAPTER 7

Reaching the Top
Election as Director of PAHO

We were at breakfast on 8 June 1993, in Santiago, Chile, when Dr Macedo said to me that I should prepare myself to succeed him. There had been tremendous speculation as to whether he would seek a fourth term. I consulted Peter Laurie, permanent secretary in the Barbados Ministry of Foreign Affairs, about the possibility of my candidature, and we agreed that it would be inappropriate for me to oppose him. One view was that the matter should be discussed with the CARICOM Heads of Government when they met in July 1993, and if they formally endorsed my candidature or even proposed that the Caribbean seek the directorship, this would absolve me of my promise not to oppose Dr Macedo. Incidentally, the view of the United States was that it would be bordering on the dishonourable to oppose Dr Macedo. At that time, we knew that Juan Manuel Sotelo, a Peruvian who was then PAHO representative in Mexico, had declared his candidature, and the Government of Peru had made formal approaches to the member governments for support. The government claimed that there was already formal support from some countries such as Mexico and one Caribbean country as well.

Dr Macedo said that he had thought of making the announcement in September at the Directing Council, but Sotelo and his government's action had precipitated his decision to speak with me. My first question was whether he would support me, to which he replied positively and promised to lobby on my behalf for Latin American support. My handwritten note to myself of that morning reads as follows:

Reaching the Top: Election as Director of PAHO

Then I started to reflect and thought about the Dunn Nutritional laboratory and other various decisions I had made in my life and wondered if I should be feeling like a reluctant bride – although no brides are really reluctant. Should I entertain self-doubt now? I will have to discuss this all with Sylvan and we will work it through together. I will have to remember to do my exercises regularly and not get too fat. But enough of this! To work! 1½ years in politics is an eternity.

I also learned that Colombia was proposing Dr Jaime Arias as a candidate. I visited Barbados on 23 June 1993 to formalize the government support and lay out a strategy with the Ministry of Foreign Affairs. I met with the prime minister, Erskine Sandiford, who had been at Mona with me. He assured me of the government's full support and that he would personally lobby his colleague heads of government. A detailed plan was prepared by the ministry, and we agreed that the campaign for this year would be centred in the Ministry of Foreign Affairs with the Ministry of Health assisting. My good friend Branford Taitt was then minister of health. There would be three phases: phase 1, immediate – up to the meeting of the CARICOM heads in July; phase 2, between July and September, which would be the date of the Directing Council meeting; and phase 3, lobbying efforts at the meeting of the Directing Council.

In discussing probable and possible support, we noted that the Caribbean might negotiate with the countries of Central America and exchange support for their candidate for the secretary general of the Organization of American States. It was also agreed that a position paper on possible changes at PAHO would not be productive, as it would give the impression that I wished to introduce radical changes to the organization. The theme would be "Continuity of Excellence". The centres of action would be the Ministry of Foreign Affairs in Barbados, and the Barbados embassy in Washington, where my friend Dr Rudi Webster was ambassador.

I was impressed with the organization of the campaign in Barbados. The ministry had a dossier on every country, with the dates of change of government, diplomatic debt to the Caribbean, and probability of support. It sent diplomatic notes to all thirty-eight countries accompanied by my curriculum vitae. The announcement of my candidacy was met with a flurry of newspaper articles in the Caribbean, pointing out not only my credentials and my suitability for the post but also the public health achievements of the region.

There was debate about the need to produce a brochure with an estimated cost of about a thousand dollars, and it was decided not to do so, partly for reasons of cost. I did prepare a non-paper on PAHO and the public's health and outlined in it the current context in terms of sociopolitical trends, the physical environment, the critical nature of information and the health and development nexus. I also outlined the areas to which PAHO would direct attention and stated that I saw our task as to see "that we build on the good and seek for the better". I said in my introduction,

> I acknowledge and laud the value of the many excellent things PAHO has done and continues to do. I am comfortable with advocating continuity of those programmes and policies that have been effective, in part because of my admiration for the administration of the current director, Dr Carlyle Guerra de Macedo, and in part because good sense indicates that I must be loyal to those policies that I myself helped to fashion and in which I acquiesced, as evidenced by my presence in the organization. My philosophy is that any change should be such as time and circumstances warrant and have clear benefit to the organization in pursuit of its proper mission and goals.

In July 1993, the Fourteenth Meeting of the Conference of CARICOM Heads of Government formally endorsed my candidature, and they all agreed to support it. I then wrote all the ministers of health asking for their support and enclosing my curriculum vitae. I learned that Juan Manuel Sotelo did so also, but while I spoke of continuity of excellence, he spoke of "a need for *change* in PAHO's Secretariat and pursuing a more effective organization with a better response capacity to the country's needs".

Just before the meeting of the Directing Council, I visited the US State Department accompanied by Ambassador Webster and met with Undersecretary Douglas Bennett and his staff. We discussed the countries from which we had received written confirmed support. There were several questions about how I would manage PAHO and what would be the major lines of technical action. They were concerned about what PAHO could do to improve management in WHO and how a new director of PAHO

Reaching the Top: Election as Director of PAHO

could promote more unity in WHO as a whole. When the issue of staff was raised, Bennett interrupted to say that as a policy, the United States would not interfere with the director's selection of staff. They would propose good people, but the choice would be that of the director. This was in contrast to the position of the Department of Health and Human Services, which wished to nominate persons to posts, specifically the post of deputy director. By the September meeting of the Directing Council, I had confirmed support from seventeen of thirty-eight countries eligible to vote. During the Directing Council, Dr Macedo invited the Latin American ministers to lunch, where my candidature was discussed. A couple of them were opposed, and doubts were expressed about my age, my lack of formal training in public health, my race, and the fear that I would Caribbeanize the organization. There was even some resistance to Dr Macedo's directness in furthering my case. During the Directing Council, I attended a reception at the Embassy of Colombia, which was still promoting Arias's candidature, and I met with the minister of health, Juan Luis Londoño, and Arias himself. They were, I think, supercilious, questioning my capacity to manage PAHO and suggesting that the candidates participate in debates in public fora throughout the Americas. Of course, I was firmly opposed to that suggestion, stating that the election was essentially a political process, and on this occasion it was fortuitous that the process would produce a competent director in myself. They were not amused.

Brazil was the first non-Caribbean country to declare its support formally, thanks no doubt to Dr Macedo's effort, and second was Chile. By 30 November 1993, there were twenty-four countries committed to me by formal communication, five or six for Arias, and three or four for Sotelo. By 17 December, there were twenty-six committed votes.

The most reluctant region was Central America, and one point of our strategy was to enlist the support of Bernardo Niehaus, who was a Costa Rican candidate for the post of secretary general of the Organization of American States and had got CARICOM support. During the World Health Assembly in Geneva in May, I met with Dr Nakajima, who expressed neutrality and then proceeded to discuss the concerns about cooperation and collaboration within WHO. He felt that there was a collegial responsibility to correct any deficiencies in WHO and expressed the hope that the new PAHO director would be cooperative in seeking a single WHO programme and policy. Of course, I agreed and promised that if I were elected, he would find in me a cooperative colleague.

In May 1994, I met with Sotelo at his request in the Miami airport. After we had exchanged pleasantries and expressions of mutual respect for one another, he proposed that we "join forces" and that Barbados should propose to Peru that he withdraw his candidature. He professed his wish to stay in PAHO, whatever the outcome of the election. I supported him in this, as I had always had high regard for him and his work. Of course, our government thought that it would be politically naive to approach Peru, granted that Barbados already had the votes for my election. In a subsequent visit to Peru, I met with the chancellor, who proposed directly that Peru would withdraw Sotelo's candidature if I agreed to nominate him as assistant director. I declined to make any commitments about staff positions.

By August 1994, I had thirty-four confirmed votes, and in a meeting in Barbados, I could discuss with Peter Laurie some aspects of management of the organization and what, if any, support I could expect and get from Barbados. We also agreed that Barbados would ask Chile to propose me, seconded by Jamaica.

The election was held on 28 September 1994, in the meeting of the Sanitary Conference. There had just been an election and a change of government in Barbados, with a new minister of health, Elizabeth Thompson, who was attending a PAHO meeting for the first time. Dr Carlos Massad, minister of health of Chile, proposed me to be the next director. He gave a résumé of my curriculum vitae, mentioning that I was a critical member of the senior management team. He said that although I was Caribbean, I had shown interest in regional matters, had learned to speak Spanish and was now an expert in the culture of the region, especially the food, the dance and the drink typical of each country. He was followed by Costa Rica, Jamaica and most of the countries present. Costa Rica proposed that the election be by acclamation, but since this was against the rules of procedure, the vote was taken, and of the thirty-eight votes cast, all were for Dr George Alleyne. This was the first time that a director had been elected for his first term unanimously.

Reaching the Top: Election as Director of PAHO

The conference then named a delegation to escort me to the conference hall comprised of Dr Macedo and representatives of every subregion: Cono Sur, Chile; Andean Region, Colombia; Central America, Costa Rica; Caribbean, Bahamas; North America, Canada.

My notes of that day include the following:

> During the voting I was surprisingly calm in my office of Assistant Director and occupied myself with reading and rereading my speech of acceptance. Sylvan was wonderful – telling me to keep calm etc. As the votes were counted and the result was 38–0 she gave me a hug and I hurried to phone my sister Cynthia. I told her that the deed was done and I was going downstairs to speak and bawl, because I could feel the emotion rising in my throat. Then five of them came to my office to get us. Massad from Chile; Weinstock from Costa Rica; Ivy Dumont of the Bahamas; Alston from Canada; Moreno from Colombia; and Carlyle. I confess that I was choked even then. As we went downstairs, Carlyle carried my speech and when we got out of the elevator, many of the staff had formed a double line through which we walked – to their cheering. When I entered the hall hand-in-hand with Sylvan, all got to their feet and applauded as we went to the dais. I was so moved: I wondered how I would get through my speech but I did. I know my voice broke a few times, but what the hell – let me have men about me who weep. When I finished they stood and applauded. If they had had sweaty caps they would like Shakespeare's Romans have flung them into the air and shouted hurrah. I would feel the waves of goodwill just washing over us.

Then the new minister from Barbados made a brilliant speech, climaxing it by proposing Dr Macedo to be director emeritus. It was an emotional occasion, and I still recall the copious weeping of the lady ministers of health of Barbados and the Bahamas at seeing a black Caribbean man reaching the pinnacle of public health in the Americas. As I took my place on the dais with my wife beside me, I confess that the film of my life to that date rolled rapidly in front of my eyes, and I indeed marvelled at the road I had trod from Lucas Street to Washington.

This is my acceptance speech, which was perhaps the finest I had given till then.

THE GROOMING OF A CHANCELLOR

You will pardon me if I read from a prepared text, but since I had some idea of the waves of emotion that would wash over me at this time, I thought it unwise to trust myself to speak without the comfort of the written word.

First, I wish to thank my own Government for having preferred my candidature and you Ministers and Heads of Delegation for having supported it. The simplicity of this thank you should not mask the deep and profound gratitude I have for you, the Representatives of the Governments of the Americas who have elected me. I am conscious of the honour you have bestowed on me and my country.

But I do not wish to dwell on honours; I would rather speak of the responsibility that comes with your mandate. I am acutely aware of the illustrious history of this Organization that has been the voice for health in our Hemisphere. I reflect with humility that I stand in a line of distinguished health professionals who have so guided its affairs that it towers tall in the world of international health.

The names of Cummins, Soper, Horwitz, Acuna and Macedo could be written on tablets that would have pride of place in any Hall of Fame of Health. There is no such hall – perhaps happily so – but the legacy of their cumulative actions is shown in even more permanent places – in the faces of men and women without pox, in the gait of children who walk without calipers or crutches.

I wish to pay tribute publicly to the Governments of Peru and Colombia. I took their presentation of candidates for the Directorship of the Pan American Health Organization as a manifestation of their concern for its well-being and a genuine and sincere desire to see that there was quality in its leadership. I am confident that I can now count on having that care and concern manifest in close cooperation and collaboration with me in the years ahead.

I would be ungrateful if at a moment like this I did not also say thanks to my wife of 36 years who has been responsible for more of my formation than she knows.

It is natural and normal to expect every new Director to speak of the changes to be introduced in his or her term of office. I am proud to have served in senior positions in the administration of Dr Carlyle Guerra de Macedo to whom I owe much, and I have the self-confidence and I am sure the agreement of this body to continue such programmes and practices that he put in place which have been successful and have done our Organization proud in the past 12 years.

Reaching the Top: Election as Director of PAHO

But Mr President, even in the continuity of which I speak there must be some modicum of change, because the times in which my predecessors were elected were different from today: the orthodoxy of our practices today was no doubt the heterodoxy of yesterday, and for sure will be the obsolescence of tomorrow. This is not the moment to enter into detail, but I believe that in order to adapt to such difference, in order to keep this Secretariat alive and responsive to the articulated needs of you in representation of the people of the Americas, it will behoove me to restate our mission, redefine the product we offer and re-engineer those parts of the management of programmes and resources that need it. It must be a management that is prudent yet innovative, one that knows how to focus and one that knows both how to subtract as well as to add as the times and circumstance warrant.

I am a product of my culture – and an integral part of that culture is our sport – our national game is cricket, a team game, whose seminal rule is fairness. In a metaphoric sense I am assuming the captaincy of a team, and I do so with a consciousness burned into me almost from birth, that captains are as good as the teams they lead. I believe that in our Secretariat we have a good team and an important, though not the only, responsibility of the leader is to bring out the best in every player and have everyone see that the final result must be greater than could be achieved by the sum of the individual efforts.

What else can you expect of me? I can promise you that in this Director you will have a person who is sensitive to the individual needs of countries, alert to the variation that exists between and within countries, and ever conscious of the standards of ethical conduct that must guide an Organization like ours. I can pledge that you will have a Secretariat that lives the motto of service – a service that is not servile, a service that is transparent, a service that is as timely and efficient as human heads and hands can make it; a service that is guided by frank and open dialogue between those who serve and those who are served. You will see your Secretariat make every effort to maintain or increase its diversity to reflect the face of our countries – diversity of sex, ethnic and national origin.

You will see your Secretariat serve all the countries of the Americas – from Baffin Bay to Cape Horn – countries large or small, continental or insular – different yes, but united in the grand design of contributing each from its strength to improving the health of all our people.

We will spare no effort; ignore no suggestion that will enhance the cohesiveness and focus of our programmes. There must be no doubt in anyone's mind that while we will continue to advocate positively or even aggressively for the understanding of the concepts of the proper place of health and for action in relation to our environment, we will not ignore the efforts that must be made to apply those health technologies that have stood the test of scientific enquiry.

I would like to think that one of the reasons you have elected me is because you share some small part or perhaps all of that vision I have of our world – one which I have articulated to some of you before. I have for a long time been gripped by a vision of a world in which there is no "otherness" in health. We may accept differences in physical characteristics – we may accept differences in ideologies – but in a very real sense, in the case of health there should be no "others", because we are indeed one, bound together by ties that go beyond our biology. For that vision to be realized, we will have to use well that most powerful of modem instruments – information – perhaps the only instrument that can close the gap between the world that is and the world that might be – the only instrument that can relieve the ignorance of many of our people who pay the cost of that ignorance in the coin of ill health and suffering. In this world that might be or will be, our citizens will truly see that health is for living and agitate that they be allowed to live in the fullest sense of the word.

I extend my hand in cooperative friendship to all the agencies, institutions and organizations that would work with us in this enormous task of assisting the peoples of the Americas in their quest for the best of health. Experience has shown me that if the goals of our countries are clearly stated and plans accurately drawn without the petty consciousness of turf that serves no purpose other than to compound inertia with ineptitude, it is possible for us to work together and achieve together.

Mr President, in a few months my name will be placed before the Executive Board of the World Health Organization to be appointed the Regional Director of that Organization for the Americas. I pledge that I will do all in my power to discharge that responsibility in such a manner as will bring credit to the Americas; I will seek to have others understand and respect the traditions and practices that have evolved over our 92 years, and hopefully contribute through sharing of knowledge and experience to ensuring that the world's health goals and objectives are achieved. I cannot in fairness

Reaching the Top: Election as Director of PAHO

speak of team spirit in the Americas and not try to translate this thinking to the global scene.

Distinguished Delegates, you have given me your support today and I ask for it during the course of my administration. With your support and counsel and with the help of the dedicated and competent band of men and women who serve their people through the Pan American Health Organization I will strive to ensure that our aspirations for the health of the Americas become realities.

And if you ask me for a bond and a surety that I will make every effort humanly possible to discharge my promises, I can only say to you, I give you my word.

PERSONAL RELATIONS

The directors who preceded me were each very different in style and in their relations with me. Dr Macedo was in my judgement a brilliant director, whom I admired and continue to admire. He had a clear grasp of the technical aspects of the organization's work and also had a remarkably political acuity. His constant affirmation that the work at the country level was where the organization produced results and his thesis that an organization like PAHO should concentrate on knowledge-work were most appropriate. In addition, he was an excellent orator, and he had the capacity to move his staff and others with his vision of what the organization could do. One of the best lessons he taught me was that it was unhelpful to criticize your predecessor, and I never heard him utter a word about the work of the organization under Dr Acuna. He had a remarkable capacity for hard work. I often marvelled at his ability to digest complicated documents in English, which was not his native language, and be able to discuss the salient aspects with clarity.

My relations with him were excellent, as they were based on mutual respect, and he would insist that if I disagreed with him and did not say so, I was doing him a disservice. We developed the practice of meeting with deputy director Robert Knouss every morning at seven-thirty when he was in Washington to discuss problems and solutions. I think he appreciated my capacity to present the problem succinctly and always with suggestions for a solution. Obviously he did not always agree with my suggested solutions, but they would be entertained seriously. I provided good staff support when we travelled together to the countries – making summaries, providing his letters of response to the issues that arose and ensuring that the relevant departments in the secretariat were kept informed of any decisions that applied to them. In particular, he made numerous references in my annual evaluations to my grasp of the essentials of organization and management.

He carried his supervision of me lightly, and we had many vigorous discussions, especially on politics and the use and abuse of power. We were always frank with one another, but, of course, this did not translate into disrespect for the office of director. I think we disagreed really fundamentally on only one occasion. He withdrew recognition that had been decided and agreed upon from a staff member in my area because of threats from a member government. This obviously damaged the pride of the staff member, who resigned immediately. This was perhaps the only occasion on which I seriously contemplated resigning, and even today I debate with myself the pros and cons of my decision to remain.

It took me some time to understand the politics of the organization while Dr Hector Acuna was director, and perhaps the predominant Latin culture made it even more problematic for me. Dr Acuna had been re-elected once, and I knew that the staff had agitated and lobbied vigorously with member governments against his re-election. It was clear he wished a third term – his predecessor, Dr Abraham Horwitz, had served four terms – but it was also clear that the feeling against him was so strong internally and among the countries that he stood little or no chance. Eventually he announced his decision not to seek a third term, claiming that he had consulted his government and asked them to let him go home to his children and grandchildren. They accepted, and therefore he would not stand again.

He was a pleasant gentleman, kind to me personally. I once invited him to lunch, and as we walked to the restaurant, he said that if "they" did not plot or intrigue against me, my future in PAHO would be bright. But he was not well liked for two reasons: his manipulation and his administrative weakness. He never seemed to have the technical details of the organization's programme at his fingertips and appeared to me to deal more in the process than in the substance of the work. But I should be grateful to him for bringing me to PAHO.

Reaching the Top: Election as Director of PAHO

I had known Dr Abraham Horwitz from a distance when I was a member of the Pan American Advisory Committee on Medical Research. He was revered by PAHO staff as an iconic director who had been responsible for much of the expansion of the organization. He was Chilean and had gained a high reputation as director of the national medical services before being elected as the first Latin American director of PAHO, where he served for four terms from 1958 to 1985. He was unsuccessful in his bid for a fifth term and during Dr Acuna's directorship maintained his office as director emeritus at the National Institutes of Health. When Dr Macedo assumed office he returned to PAHO and was a remarkable and enjoyable source of information and inspiration to myself and the many staff members with whom he interacted.

I never ceased to marvel at his recall of detail. He would tell of the growth of the organization during his tenure, how its budget increased by over fifty per cent to almost US$50 million and the staff to almost fifteen hundred, the majority of whom were in the field. This was when the Caribbean countries gained independence and joined the organization. He was especially proud of PAHO's advocacy for the role of health in alleviating much of the poor social and economic conditions of the Americas, as he took very seriously PAHO's constitutional responsibility "to combat disease, lengthen life and promote the physical and mental health of the people".

He had been convinced of the role of human resources as key to the administration of the region's health services and would regale me the details of the formation of the Pan American Health and Education Foundation (of which he was then president) and the loan negotiated from the Inter-American Development Bank for a programme to provide inexpensive education materials for Latin American students. His dream of a Latin American university had been unrealized and he hinted that perhaps I would undertake the challenge.

I recall particularly a discussion with him on PAHO's role in non-democratic countries and he was emphatic that the organization should maintain a presence in the country irrespective of the political regime. He smiled as he said that one of the things of which he was not proud was the fact that PAHO had given the Haitian dictator Dr François Duvalier a fellowship to pursue his master's degree in public health at Johns Hopkins University. But that was before he became a dictator.

It was during his tenure as director that the organization had moved to its present location and it was in large measure due to his negotiating skills that most of the funding came as an interest-free mortgage from the W.K. Kellogg Foundation. He continued to be actively involved in international nutrition almost up to the time of his death in 2000 at age eighty-nine.

THE TRANSITION

I was elected in September 1994 but would not assume office until 1 February 1995. This hiatus relates to the relationship between PAHO and WHO. I was elected by the governments of the Americas to be director of the Pan American Sanitary Bureau but would need to be appointed by the executive board of WHO in January 1995 to be the director of the Regional Office of WHO in the Americas. The interval of four months could have posed some difficulty, as I continued in my position as assistant director and set about making plans to manage the organization when I assumed the directorship. Luckily for me, Dr Macedo was magnificent. He made no major decision in this interval without consulting me and discussed with me many of the problems that were likely to occur, especially those related to the budget.

I reread recently my handwritten notes of December 1994, in which I recorded some of the ideas I considered during the period of transition. I had lunch with Dr Acuna, who advised me to concentrate on specific programmes and short-term goals, as politicians would only appreciate and support these. He said that it was useful conceptually to have a long vision and to see PAHO as a development agency, but in practice this is not the lens through which politicians view health. Of course, I demurred, as I believed that health would not be improved by concentrating only on those issues that traditionally lay within the purview of the health sector. I would say to myself, *He knows not health who only health knows.*

The notion of a transition itself intrigued me. I know there was a view that transitions begin with an ending and that it is necessary to let go of current practices if there is to be progress. Part of the trauma of transition or change comes from breaking with the current situation. This was the order of nature. The leaves fall; winter comes before the spring. I instinctively rejected that perception and regarded the transition as a period of building upon what went before. It should be a period for continuing the good practices and introducing any change in an evolutionary manner.

Among my notes was the injunction to avoid like the plague the use of the Spanish expression *se debe*, meaning "one ought to". I felt that this should never be used in PAHO but should be replaced with a more positive "we will" or "we can", both of which accepted responsibility and did not leave action to some vague other. I entertained the concept of a chief of staff and rejected it, believing that my office could function perfectly well with competent administrative and secretarial staff – as indeed it did.

I reflected on the role of extra budgetary funding on the organization and determined that such funds would always be dedicated to the established priorities as set out by our governing bodies, and PAHO should not be held hostage to the particular interests of a country or individual or granting agency. I determined to expunge the word *donor* from our lexicon. It was common to speak of donor funds and set out classifications of different categories of donors. I would insist on regarding them as partners rather than donors and would say that in PAHO, we would only accept partners and that at least in terms of countries, they were all donors, and all were recipients. The smaller countries would not give as much in material things, and they might contribute with ideas rather than money, but they were valuable nonetheless. As for external funding, I would propose that this be in the nature of a partnership, not a donor–recipient relationship. I knew this view was not universal in WHO.

On a more domestic level, I determined to strengthen the office of the person responsible for advising new staff on their arrival in Washington. I felt that no new staff member could really do his or her work if there was confusion and uncertainty about settling, housing, schooling and the many domestic pieces of a new life in a strange place.

I selected a transition team from among some senior staff with whom I discussed various programmatic and organizational issues. Many of my colleagues assumed that there would be major changes in direction and personnel, and there was intense lobbying for various positions. The concept of organizational re-engineering was very much in vogue, having been popularized partly by the attention given to it by the vice president of the United States, Al Gore. I had read fairly widely on re-engineering as applied to business and decided that the basic thesis and the method did not apply to an organization like ours.[1] I did not see the need for a fundamental shift in the focus of our activities on improving health in the member countries or that our basic business model was intrinsically flawed. I was also concerned that some of the examples seemed to create chaos before rebuilding the organization according to some new paradigm. I explained to the team that service organizations like PAHO change better by evolution than by revolution, and discontinuity in our work that would accompany revolutionary change would be extremely disruptive. There was no need for the major structural repositioning of the organization, which seemed to be an essential prerequisite of the re-engineering process, and in addition, many of the concepts that applied to business did not apply to PAHO. We were not in competition for market share, and although globalization obviously affected us, it did not impinge materially on the direction of our work, at least in the short term.

One corollary of the decision to manage change in an evolutionary way was that there was no need to employ change managers or change agents, and more emphasis was placed on organizational development that implied mobilizing staff to adhere to and buy in to a vision which they helped to create. Thus an organization-wide process was begun to create a vision and mission statement for us. I emphasized to the team that the country offices would remain the critical point of interaction with governments for the delivery of our technical cooperation, but the central or regional offices would not be appendages of the country offices. It would be necessary to outline clearly the functions pertaining to the different levels of the organization, which I did.

There was considerable discussion about a possible new structure, but I made it clear that the structure of the organization was an expression of the philosophy and management style of the director, and the basic rule of "structure following function" would apply. It must reflect the possibility of operationalizing what I considered the two essential value principles which would guide the organization during my term of office – equity and pan-Americanism. I will refer to these again. I settled on a bureaucratic divisional structure which to me would embody a hierarchy of responsibilities, clear definition of roles and an efficient evaluation system that could enhance performance. During the last years of Dr Macedo's administration, he had organized some of the programme activities to incorporate some elements of Demming's quality circles and emphasize cross-programmatic planning. The idea was excellent, but in my view, it had not been optimally successful for many reasons intrinsic to the nature of the programmes and perhaps the cultural characteristics of the staff.

I was comfortable with an organization that had staff and line responsibilities. I was aware of the conflicts that were common between staff and line offices and their managers and was equally aware that the management of these conflicts depended greatly on the personnel, the conflict management style of the senior staff and the quality of supervision. I saw the line divisions as being responsible primarily for the technical output of the organization and the staff offices being predominantly advisory. I say predominantly, because given the nature of our work, there would be overlaps on occasion, as PAHO provided advice at the country level in areas that might theoretically fall within the purview of the staff offices. But as in any organization, the functioning of the structure would depend in large measure on other aspects of the management style of the leader.

One of my first tests was in the selection of the deputy and assistant directors. The deputy traditionally had been an American, and I believe that this was proper given the fact that the United States paid the lion's share of our budget. I went to see the assistant secretary of state for Latin American Affairs, and he said quite bluntly again that the naming of the deputy was my choice. The responsibility for the secretariat was mine, and therefore I had to be comfortable with my deputy. There was lobbying from other parts of the US government for various candidates, and the actual deputy, Robert Knouss, wished to continue. I decided to appoint David Brandling-Bennett, who was then head of the communicable disease programme, because I had been impressed by his forthrightness and his grasp of the problems in his area.

For the post of assistant director, I appointed Mirta Roses, an Argentinian who was then PAHO representative in Bolivia. She was flabbergasted when I called her, and her reaction was "Why me?" I was aware that her compatriot, Luis Argentino Pico, sub-secretary for health in Argentina, felt that he was the most qualified person for the position, as he had been an ardent participant in our governing bodies and had the support of his minister. I appointed Mirta because as her supervisor as assistant director, I had been impressed by her competence, her fearlessness, her willingness to express her opinion, her interpersonal skills, and in addition, I wished to promote women in the organization. To put it mildly, the minister of health of Argentina, Dr Alberto Mazza, was not pleased, and over lunch in Buenos Aires, he asked why I did not consult him if I wished to have an Argentinian in that position in the organization. I listened and then explained to him gently that the decision was mine, and I had to be comfortable with the person I appointed. It is a decision that I have never regretted – to the contrary, she proved to be outstanding in the position.

CHAPTER 8

The Office of Director
Assumption of Office

The first surprise for many staff was that I retained all of the personnel in my office, including my driver. I made it clear that our relationship would be one of trust, respect and loyalty, but they would be subsumed under loyalty to the organization and its principles. This approach was criticized by some staff initially, especially those from the Latin countries, some of whom were accustomed to wholesale shifts of personnel with the advent of a new administration. One staff member quipped in jest that he had expected even the lady who served coffee would be changed.

In my initial address on installation I retraced some of the history of the organization, recalling the signing of the Pan American Sanitary Code in 1925 – the formal treaty that sustained the organization, emphasizing that the code was an agreement among equals, and the organization "was designed to facilitate the working of this joint venture of equals seeking to do together that which each could not do alone". I emphasized that PAHO had to be a champion of the search for equity and social justice that found expression in Health for All.

The concept of equity remained fundamental to our work. My concern for equity had perhaps been born out of my understanding of the concept from Aristotle's ethics that equals must be treated equally and unequals must be treated unequally. I had sometimes referred to this principle vulgarly as "the greatest form of inequality is to treat unequals equally". The concept as applied in health relates mainly to the differences in one or other health measure between peoples which is unfair and beyond the volition of the less favoured. Thus in health it is given a moral cloak, as there is no reason intrinsic to being human why there should be avoidable health differentials. The essential search then must be to detect the differences and put in place the appropriate mechanisms for reducing the inequality. Obviously there are inequalities that do not qualify as being inequitable. The concept has been parsed in various ways – for example, differences are made between horizontal and vertical equity. The former implies equal treatment of equals, while the latter indicates that there should be unequal treatment of unequals. I often contend that this is simply a restatement of Aristotle's basic thesis.

I took the view that one could measure inequality and then impute inequity, but *sensu strictu*, there was no way that one could measure inequity, given that it was impossible to quantify the moral aspect. There are several measures of inequality, and the difference between simple averages could be amplified by measures such as concentration curves and derivations of indices similar to the Gini coefficient so beloved by economists.

The focus on equity had several programmatic implications for PAHO. It meant that there had to be emphasis on measuring the health status of populations, and such measurements had to move beyond national averages to disaggregation by groups and location, for example. It was critical in determining inequity to be clear about the stratifiers to be used. Some of them were binary, such as gender, while others were ordinal or would have scales or gradients such as income or educational level. I often referred to the tyranny of the national averages which hid the situation of people in one or other disadvantaged group. It was often revealing to find that within countries in which the national average for some indicator was appropriately high or low and was a cause for celebration or congratulation, there were several marginalized groups which could only be detected when the data were disaggregated by the appropriate stratifier. The second major implication was the focus of attention and programmes on those for whom the scales had been weighted disadvantageously.

The notion of a pan-American approach was not new. I would quote Elihu Root, a former US secretary of state, who in an address to a pan-American congress in Rio de Janeiro in 1906 said, "No nation can live unto itself alone and continue to live. Each nation's growth is a part of the development of the race. There may be leaders and there may be laggards, but no nation can long continue very far in advance of the general progress of mankind and no nation that is not doomed to extinction can remain very far behind." These sentiments were, of course, in relation to the attention being paid to Latin America by President Theodore Roosevelt, given the opening of the Panama Canal, which was possibly an instrument of division among the American states.

Although pan-Americanism has sometimes been regarded suspiciously as a mask for the hegemony of the United States, in contemporary terms it meant for me coordinated effort by the countries of the Americas to address their health problems and concern by the better off for the situation of the less well endowed.[1] There had already been spectacular progress in eradicating smallpox, and the Americas were well on the way to being certified as having eliminated poliomyelitis. But it was not only in infectious diseases that there was room for a pan-American approach to health.

In my speech on election I had said that we would traffic in information, and I saw that one of the strengths of PAHO lay in the use of such information. I cited T.S. Eliot as he invoked the endless cycle of idea and action.[2]

> Where is the life we have lost in living?
> Where is the wisdom we have lost in knowledge?
> Where is the knowledge we have lost in information?

And Harlan Cleveland would add, "Where is the information we have lost in data?"[3] I believe in the hierarchy of data, information, knowledge and wisdom. It is the information that was our stock and trade. It is that transportable and indestructible resource that is transmitted to individuals who internalize it and integrate it with other information, thus acquiring knowledge of the senses and of the mind. It is the wisdom derived from knowledge refined that forms the basis of most human action. For as his minister said to the Yellow Emperor in the Nei Ching[4] as they spoke of unity, "When the minds of the people are closed and wisdom is locked out they remain tied to disease."

This emphasis on information would be translated to the structure of the organization, as I believed that information has to be the most important element in a structure like ours, which has so many sub-systems. I established the Special Program for Health Situation Analysis, which published annually a set of basic health indicators of the Americas. I would emphasize that the situation analysis and interpretation of information related to the health of our member states was part of the constitutional responsibility of PAHO. The practice of publishing basic health indicators on a regular basis was taken up by other regions of the WHO. This special programme collaborated with countries in establishing health situation rooms containing updated health information to be used as a planning tool and not merely as a static record. In addition, PAHO published every four years a major opus on the health situation in the Americas, complete with commentaries on the important health issues in every country. This was recognized and widely cited as the best source of information on health in the region.

There was a unit responsible for producing the scientific and technical information for which PAHO had rightly become well known and respected. PAHO almost from its inception had given prominence to the publication of scientific information, and the *Boletin Panamericano de Salud* was one of the region's oldest public health journals. We would provide information to our various publics about what was being done by PAHO and with PAHO. This would be public information, broadly speaking, and would involve our media coverage throughout the Americas. Finally, we had to have robust internal information systems that kept track of the use of our resources, human and financial, as transparency was of critical importance in an organization that was responsible to thirty-eight governments.

There was a separate unit for planning and analysis that was responsible for developing the organization's planning and evaluation instruments, and the head of that unit served as secretary of the director's cabinet. I took the view that budgeting was properly a part of finance, although I was aware of the rationale for combining planning and budgeting in one unit.

MANAGEMENT OF THE ORGANIZATION

I have never taken any formal classes in management or organizational theory, and my interest in these was sparked in a peculiar way. One day

The Office of Director: Assumption of Office

while I was engaged in research in the Tropical Metabolism Research Unit in the 1960s, Sylvan, who was then enrolled in the social work programme at the University of the West Indies, brought home a slender volume entitled *Bureaucracy in Modern Society* by Peter Blau.[5] I began to read it, becoming fascinated and a little concerned. I realized that in the fullness of time I would have to manage an organization, and I had no clue as to how they operated. I had the popular negative view of bureaucracy and was intrigued to learn from Blau that a bureaucratic organization was one designed to accomplish large-scale tasks by systematically coordinating the work of many individuals. Bureaucracy then was intended to improve organizational efficiency. I was intrigued by the clarity with which Blau set out the four factors that characterized a bureaucratic organization. These were specialization, a hierarchy of authority, a system of rules, and impersonality. I would appreciate later the difference between bureaucracy and what I would call "bureaupathology", which occurs when the bureaucratic process is perverse and becomes an end in itself. There is ritualistic observance of rules and regulations, and the hierarchy becomes a source of corruption.

I then set myself to read widely about management and organizational theory and behaviour. Peter Drucker was my guru originally,[6] and I became enthusiastic about the operation of systems and the extent to which in small societies and organizations with limited resources and open to a variety of shocks, one could indeed manage by objective. In my first years in PAHO, I read more intensively about various theories of management and saw the possibilities of applying some of these principles I had learned to my work. It became increasingly clear, however, that much of the literature dealt with for-profit organizations, and I found little or nothing related to intergovernmental structures.

There are many differences between these two types of organizations, but I will highlight only two of them here. In the for-profit organization, it is easy to quantify and value the outputs and outcomes. This is not possible in the intergovernmental organizations, and there is no system of material rewards linked to effort or outcome. Second, there is no system of automatic promotion with or as a result of increased responsibility. In the for-profit organizations and similarly in a university system to which I was accustomed, there was the expectation of promotion based on performance. In the intergovernmental organizations, a professional is hired to carry out a specific set of tasks to which a specific grade is attached, and there is no mechanism for promotion through the bureaucracy based on performance. Of course, there are examples of persons starting at a low level and rising to the top. Kofi Anann is the classic example of this. He entered the United Nations as a P4 and eventually became secretary general. In such cases, it is institutional politics that play the major role in smoothing the path for promotion. It is for this reason that I advise young people to enter these organizations when they have had national experience, are mature and so confident in themselves that they do not look for automatic advancement based on performance. But also, because of the nature of the indicators of performance, it was almost impossible to release an individual, although there may be widespread acknowledgement of poor performance.

TECHNICAL COOPERATION

When I entered PAHO, it struck me that there was considerable imprecision as regards the exact nature of its work. I would question the essence of our output and would often cite what I understood to be a cardinal rule of business: "Know your public; know your product." PAHO's staff had intimate knowledge of the member countries and when questioned about their activities would offer as a reply that they "worked with countries" to support various programmes. I found remarkable reverence for the documents produced in the resolutions of the governing bodies, as if these were substantial products of the organization, although I could find little systematic evaluation of the degree to which these resolutions were followed. PAHO's staff were excellent professionals, the vast majority of them technically superb and well versed in their disciplines. Most of them came from the best and most prestigious universities of the Americas. I must insist here that this does not in any way detract from the tremendous effort made by the dedicated PAHO staff at all levels to seek to address the major health problems of the countries. I developed and retain tremendous respect for the technical skill and dedication of PAHO staff, who would go to great lengths, often at personal sacrifice, to try to alleviate these problems.

The Office of Director: Assumption of Office

In the university, the product was clear. We were committed to teaching, research and service, and all three of these could be measured. Although we struggled with pedagogical evaluation and often argued when some professorial appointment was questioned, because the major accomplishment of the person proposed was excellence in teaching, there was some general agreement on what that meant. In addition, we could point to the numbers of graduates and the research papers published and could itemize our service. But I found it difficult to determine PAHO's major product, and I became increasingly dissatisfied with the weakness of our ability to be more precise about the meaning of technical cooperation. So I set myself to read about what I considered the actual work of PAHO, and over the years invested considerable personal effort in systematizing it. This was not the effort or thinking of a single person, and much is owed to the input of Dr Macedo as director and two other staff members – Juan Manuel Sotelo and Lily Hidalgo.

Cooperation had been the leitmotif of the very foundation of PAHO – an organization that was born out of the desire of the countries of the Americas to cooperate in addressing mainly the problems of infectious disease. The major sources of concern initially were yellow fever and cholera. The activities to be carried out were conceived as cooperative ones among equal sovereign states. Thus, in the preamble to the Sanitary Code of 1924, which is the formal treaty that created and legitimizes the organization, the founding governments "entered into a convention to the end that effective cooperative international measures may be applied for the prevention of the international spread of the communicable infections of human beings".

There were numerous attempts pre-Second World War to develop cooperative mechanisms in international health, and the most noticeable example of this was the International Office of Public Health, a creature of the League of Nations to which the United States never subscribed. In the post-bellum era, there was an acute consciousness of the need for cooperation for peace and by extension for health, as there were tragic consequences of the isolationism that had characterized much of the period between the wars. The United Nations that was born of that need incorporated into its charter "cooperation in solving international problems of an economic, social, cultural or humanitarian character".

I believe that the emphasis for international cooperation in social affairs was sparked in part by President Truman in his famous inaugural address in January 1949: "For the first time in history, humanity possesses the knowledge and the skill to relieve the suffering of these people." These words still remain for me some of the most noble expressions of man's desire to help the less fortunate. I do not neglect the possibility of self-interest, but it is possible to read into them a large dose of sheer altruism and the magnanimity that I have always wished to believe came from a genuine humanist. But there is a clear distinction to be drawn between cooperation among nation-states – international cooperation – and the help given by one nation or by intergovernmental organizations to another nation. The term espoused by WHO in making these benefits available was technical assistance. Experts from the developed countries would assist their counterparts in the poor countries. The notion was very much that of the rich helping the poor, and the dominant concept was one of messianic assistance. The United Nations systematically classified its technical assistance as providing expert advice through international experts, equipment and supplies, and training persons from the developing countries. Indeed, according to WHO's constitution, one of its functions was "to furnish technical assistance and in emergencies necessary aid upon the request or acceptance of governments".

Incidentally, the international system did not initially conceive of the possibility of experts from developing countries rendering assistance to others, but in WHO, and certainly PAHO when I entered, the majority of the staff was from developing countries. Over time it became clear that the term *assistance* bordered on the pejorative, and the nature of international work was more in keeping with cooperation, that is, working with persons in the developing countries as partners. Indeed, in 1977, WHO formally rejected the concept of technical assistance that implied a donor–recipient relationship and replaced it with technical cooperation, which was founded on "the common and mutual interest of all, whereby member states cooperate with their Organization, as equal partners, to define and achieve their health goals through programmes that are determined by their needs and priorities and that promote their self-reliance in health development". But no one could tell me the elements of that cooperation.

I analysed the various activities carried out by PAHO's staff over a period of six years and developed a taxonomy of our technical cooperation. This was important, as the term itself is not self-defining, and the term and what it implies were interpreted differently by different organizations. For example, international financing organizations tended to define it purely in monetary terms, usually loans and the expenditure that accompanied them. I could now propose that this taxonomy be used as the basis of our programming.[7] The six strategic approaches of the technical cooperation were described as (1) resource mobilization, (2) dissemination of information, (3) training, (4) development of norms, plans and policies, (5) promotion of research, and (6) provision of direct technical consultation. I was amused when I was told on visiting one of our offices that I was referred to affectionately as "Taxonomy George". Our thesis indeed was that the concept of cooperation was intrinsic to the organization itself. The effectiveness of the programme of technical cooperation is enhanced by a system of planning, programming and evaluation (AMPES–AMRO Programming and Evaluation System), which had been developed long before I became director.

One of the advantages of attempting to objectivize and codify our technical cooperation was that it made it easier to explain to newcomers exactly what they should do. Incoming technical staff often had the illusion that their job was to carry out programmes in the member countries – to kill the mosquitoes themselves. It was sometimes difficult to convince them that their job was not to kill the mosquitoes but to assist the countries to put in place the policies, plans and programmes to kill the mosquitoes.

The second development in this regard was a change in the notion of technical cooperation among developing countries (TCDC) itself. The decade of the 1970s saw increasing anticolonial feeling and growth of the notion that the world's affairs were dominated by a group of rich industrial countries. The whole international system was in a state of flux, out of which arose the call for a new international economic order. There was a loud demand for technical and economic cooperation among developing countries and the development of self-sufficiency in them. It was in this atmosphere that a landmark conference on TCDC was held in 1978 in Buenos Aires, which developed a detailed plan of action for that cooperation.[8] The first objective was as follows: "To foster the self-reliance of developing countries through the enhancement of their creative capacity to find solutions to their development problems in keeping with their own aspirations values and special needs." One parallel declaration went as far as to declare boldly that "TCDC is a historical imperative brought about by the need for a new international order".[9]

It was natural and logical for health to be cast within this concept of TCDC globally and regionally, and PAHO convened two working groups on TCDC in health in 1983 and 1984. There was intense discussion in the governing bodies, with several resolutions providing mandates for promoting the concept and practice of TCDC. The United Nations even established a fund in 1983 with the specific purpose of supporting technical and economic cooperation activities among developing countries of the Group of 77.

I was perhaps the person who argued most vigorously and convinced the director that PAHO should focus on technical cooperation among all countries, and that the concept of technical cooperation only among the developing countries was pejorative, obsolete and contrary to the spirit and logic behind the establishment of PAHO itself.[10] The notion of pan-Americanism enshrined the concept of equality among nations – at least of the Americas.

I contended that there should be cooperation among all countries, and the role of PAHO would be to provide technical cooperation to the individual countries and to foster and support technical cooperation among the countries themselves (TCC). The sequence of events for the development of PAHO's technical cooperation should be: to (1) identify national priorities; (2) identify the need for technical cooperation; (3) identify the need for that technical cooperation to be satisfied by PAHO; and (4) formulate the technical cooperation programme. It was clear that any need for TCC would be formulated at the same time that PAHO and the country identified the overall need for technical cooperation.

In our initial systematic search for examples of technical cooperation at the country level, we found that health was not a prominent component of that cooperation, with one marked exception. Cuba had made such cooperation a part of its health and foreign policy, and the placement of Cuban health professionals in other developing countries was a classic example

The Office of Director: Assumption of Office

of TCC. It was sometimes alleged that this was more in the nature of a commercial enterprise than TCC, but I do know of examples in which there was no financial consideration.

The responsibility of such TCC as there was, usually resided in the ministries of foreign affairs. There were usually no focal points in the ministries of health, and in general there was a lack of information and perhaps enthusiasm for TCC in health at the country level. However, PAHO could point out that its regional centres were examples of TCC. Several aspects of the subregional health initiatives represented this form of cooperation, and the initiative in the Caribbean – the Caribbean Cooperation in Health – by its very name indicated that its fundamental base was TCC.

In a meeting convened by WHO in Jakarta in 1993, Juan Manuel Sotelo and I argued forcibly for the change in focus from TCDC to TCC.[11] Although our WHO colleagues accepted the logic of our proposals, there was less than enthusiasm for changing their thinking and practice.[12]

The focal point for overseeing the country technical cooperation programmes fell within the office of the assistant director, and when I occupied that position, I was responsible for formulating more precisely the processes to be undertaken for developing and funding specific TCC projects. I would insist that the modalities of technical cooperation that I had elaborated as a taxonomy were generic and applicable to all forms of technical cooperation in health, including TCC. The United Nations would still persist with the concept of TCDC, although in a review in 1997 it was noted that south–south cooperation – a euphemism for TCDC – should not be considered a substitute for north–south cooperation, and triangular approaches should be considered. There appeared to be reluctance to accept the notion that south–south cooperation really marched to a political ideological drum and that the constitution of the United Nations mandated it to promote cooperation among all countries. I view the current effort to resuscitate the notion that there is some intrinsic value to south–south cooperation as anachronistic at best and pejorative at worse. Similarly, the notion of triangular cooperation is limited. The idea should be one of cooperation among all the countries of the world with the inputs coming from wherever they can most appropriately be sourced.

After I became director, the responsibility for overseeing TCC still remained with the assistant director, under whom the approach of TCC was well coordinated and made a point for evaluation within the rubric of the evaluation of the country programmes. I increased significantly the funds for TCC, which were specifically allotted in addition to the regular country budgets, and a financing mechanism was designed expressly to track them. There was perceptible growth in the number of TCC projects and increasing acceptance by the countries of TCC as a useful adjunct to the cooperation from PAHO or from other sources. I saw it as another expression of pan-Americanism,[13] and I would insist that all the countries contributed or had the capacity to contribute to the collective effort to improve health in the Americas. The programme of TCC at the country level was strengthened and expanded under Mirta Roses as assistant director.

DECISION-MAKING

Most of the basic principles of effective decision-making apply in an international organization. First, there is the need for data capture, gathering the necessary information and rinsing it with the appreciation of the giver of the information. In international organizations the material stakes are small; thus there is tremendous importance placed on personal recognition, so much of the information given is tinged with the possibility of personal advantage. The nature of the organization and the importance of information as a tool to gain personal advantage do not contribute to a culture of sharing information. But as I have discovered, this applies in international organizations in general and is not unique to PAHO.

Dr Macedo had established an advisory committee which usually met monthly. I continued this practice but named the committee my "cabinet" and tried to have it function according to my appreciation of the nature of the Westminster parliamentary model. It comprised the deputy and assistant directors, chief of administration, and the heads of the divisions, with the Office of Planning serving as the secretary. There were some differences, however, between the Westminster model and mine. The director was not really *primus inter pares* – he was primus! I recall reference to the circular table around which we sat and some wag posting a cartoon of a new member enquiring where was the head of the table. The answer was, "Wherever the boss sits, that is the head." I would entertain discussion and debate with the firm belief that they were essential to making good decisions. But there was one feature which sometimes infuriated some of my colleagues. I would insist that there would be no "free" conversation with the more aggressive making their contributions by intervening whenever they saw fit. I would insist that persons indicate when they wished to speak, be recognized and then speak. I was accused of being a schoolmaster, but I was convinced that this was the best way of garnering the opinion of the group and then being able to synthesize the discussion and reach a conclusion that could be minuted.

The invitation of multiple comments often meant that items took a long time, which was sometimes a source of frustration, but I genuinely believed that participation was essential if there was going to be ownership of the decision. I cannot say that I was always in agreement with the collective decision, but that was never about matters I considered essential or critical, and I never invested my persona in a decision. Once a decision was taken, my style was to move on and not agonize unduly if it was correct or not. Given the opportunities for monitoring and evaluation, the decision could be changed eventually if necessary.

Decision-making in decentralized organizations brings its challenges, and one is to ensure that individuals in the decentralized units accept and follow the decisions taken. I embraced the concept of due process for making global strategies work.[14] In practical terms, due process meant the following: that the central office is familiar with the situation in the decentralized units; that two-way communication is possible in the decision-making process; that there is consistency in decision-making across the decentralized units; that the decentralized units can challenge the decisions made; and that the decentralized units receive an explanation for the process and outcome of the decision-making.

All minutes of the cabinet meetings were distributed to the offices and centres, and during my visits, I encouraged staff in these offices to be familiar with and query if necessary the decisions we took. On several occasions I received telephone calls from our representatives questioning one or other of the decisions taken in cabinet.

Consistency in decision-making is one of the more critical elements for all organizations, and I will give one example. I had decided that I would never appoint someone from outside the organization to be a PAHO/WHO representative in a country office, as I had seen unfortunate results of such appointments. I often referred to the organization of the Roman Empire. This is not an exact parallel, but it suffices. I would ask why they were no revolts that threatened Imperial Rome, which originated in the provinces. Why did the Roman consul in Judea never mobilize his legions and attack Rome? How did Rome manage its empire without faxes and emails? My answer was that the consul was socialized into being Roman before he left Rome for Judea and did not need faxes or emails to instruct him how to act as a good Roman. I was firm in my belief that our representatives had to be socialized into being PAHO staff before being sent to head a country office.

On one occasion, the ambassador from a major country came to see me with a message from his president. The president wished me to appoint an ex-minister of health as a representative in a neighbouring country, and he gave me the assurance that any objections would be removed by agreements at the presidential level. I demurred and then rejected the request, explaining the principle which I followed in appointing representatives. The ambassador was furious, threatening me and the organization with dire retribution. This was not a trivial matter, but I made the decision stand and subsequently had to negotiate away the ill feeling that obviously had arisen. There was an interesting follow-up to that incident. Years later I went to that country to be honoured with one of its highest awards, and that ambassador who had now returned to the Ministry of Foreign Affairs was the one to place the sash over my shoulder and present the medal to be given to me by the minister. We did not even recognize one another!

MANAGING DIVERSITY

When I began to read about organizational management, especially in the United States, the aspect of encouraging diversity was prominent. It seemed that the move was away from affirmative action to managing diversity, as diverse workforces were more productive, and in addition, diversity was a matter of morality and decency. There were two aspects that occupied my thinking. First, there was the position of women in the organization. This was a matter of concern throughout WHO, and there were several reasons given for not having women in the professional ranks, and the consequence was therefore not having them in senior positions. The reason or excuse in Africa, for example, was that the educational systems which disadvantaged girls meant that there were fewer women available for professional posts. A reason put forward in the Americas was the macho culture, which made it difficult for men to be the trailing spouses. This had been recognized by my predecessor, but I decided that PAHO should make a more aggressive effort to incorporate and promote women. It was just the right thing to do.

I would recall the opinion of Sir Arthur Lewis, former principal and vice chancellor of the University of the West Indies, in regard to the need to have more West Indians on staff. The argument was often put forward that the West Indian might be qualified to do the job, but there were others better qualified than he or she. But Sir Arthur instructed that once the West Indian was qualified, he or she should be appointed, as suitability was often in the eye of the beholder. For several years, I insisted that once the female applicant was qualified to do the job, she should have preference. I also appreciated the importance of selection committees and remarked once in jest that "if a selection committee is composed of cockroaches then your staff will be predominantly cockroaches". Thus the rule was that there could be no selection for a post unless a quarter of the applicants were women, and every selection committee must include women. I was pleased to see the number of women in the higher professional posts increasing during my term of office, and as I have noted before, I was pleased to appoint a woman as assistant director and have her succeed me as director. She was the first woman to head a regional office in WHO.

But there are other aspects of diversity. There is cultural sensitivity over what I would call the integrity of the persona. One had to be careful about comments related to a person's work that might be interpreted as diminishing the persona. I recall a comical aspect to this appreciation of cultural diversity. In the Anglo-Saxon milieu, there is considerable respect for the integrity of personal space. Persons shake hands, and public displays of affection are not the norm. But I discovered in PAHO that kissing ladies in public, on the cheek, of course, and embracing them was a normal greeting.

So after a few years I found myself adopting or adapting to these practices and would freely kiss and hug ladies on greeting them. When I became director, an American female member of staff sent me an email, or it might have been a telephone call, expressing the hope that I would desist from the practice of hugging and kissing female staff. I immediately desisted, but a couple weeks later, some Latin ladies commented to me that since I was now director, I had become standoffish and impersonal, and perhaps thought I was now too good to kiss and greet them affectionately. Everyone cannot be pleased, so I reverted happily to hugging and kissing ladies to the satisfaction of most – or at least, so I believe.

EVALUATION

Programme evaluation is an integral part of the cybernetic cycle of planning, programming, implementation, evaluation, correction, planning. Evaluation was well developed in PAHO, and there was at least one staff member in the Division of Human Resources with considerable expertise in summative and formative evaluation for specific programmes. When I became area director, it was clear to me that there was need for a more formal annual programme evaluation. Initially my area and then progressively the whole organization carried out annual evaluations. I had been convinced of the value of evaluation of social programmes from the work of Carol Weiss but believed many of our programmes were not evaluable according to the criteria of evaluability.[15] Parenthetically, some senior PAHO staff were philosophically opposed to evaluation, with one describing it as contrary to human nature. In rebuttal, I would contend that the fact that comparative adjectives existed in most languages meant that humans were wedded to evaluation, comparison implying prior evaluation. He was not convinced. But good evaluation implies that the programme as designed is evaluable, and evaluability assessment should figure prominently in programme development.

There was another significant development at this time which advanced the theory and practice of programme evaluation in the organization. PAHO adopted the logical framework for its programming. Much of this was spearheaded by Lily Hidalgo working in the Office of Strategic

Planning. In essence the logical framework as we applied it allowed staff to set project objectives; define indicators of success; identify key activity groups; define critical assumptions; and identify means of verification and defined resources required for implementation. I promoted the link between evaluation and the logical framework, but the main weakness in the process was that it was impossible, given the nature of our budget organization, to define and allot all the resources necessary for implementation. The logical framework probably has been overtaken by other systems for project design and management, but it served its purpose for a time, forcing staff into more precision, and defining the proposed outputs, the levels of responsibility and the outcome of the technical cooperation.

Programme evaluation in an organization should be complemented with personnel evaluation. The system I inherited was arcane, did not allow for objective evaluation of performance and did not provide for adequate and timely input of the supervisor into the work of the supervised. We set about refining the system into an eventual personal performance evaluation system in which the supervisor and supervised established jointly the work objectives for the period. At the end of it is a joint revision by both with the purpose of assessing the degree to which the objectives have been met and, in case of non-achievement of results, the manner in which a supervisor can assist. Ideally the system is designed to assist staff in achieving their full potential and not merely in defining non-achievement or being punitive.

CHAPTER 9

A New International Challenge
The Director General of the World Health Organization

The candidature for the post of director general of the World Health Organization has to be one of the most fascinating lessons in international politics that I ever experienced. Since Dr Nakajima's re-election as director general for a second term in 1993, there had been growing dissatisfaction with his management of the organization. From this distance, it is clearer how this arose, and it was fuelled by the many interests within and without WHO. First, however, I must state that my personal relations with Dr Nakajima were cordial, and he respected me and in several instances supported my management of PAHO. Of course, there were differences which often arose in meetings of senior staff, which included the regional directors, and the deputy and assistant directors, with regard to programming and politics, but this is normal in any organization. These were never major, but I could understand how the management style could cause dissatisfaction among the member states. He was a man of wide tastes and interests. He read the scientific literature avidly and was one of the few persons I know who read the prestigious journals *Nature* and *Science* regularly and could converse intelligently about their contents. He was knowledgeable on a diverse range of subjects and often surprised audiences by expounding on subjects as diverse as the Argentinian tango, Australian wines and Persian carpets. I recall one such experience. I met with him in Buenos Aires after I had visited some Andean countries, includ-

A New International Challenge: The Director General of the WHO

ing Bolivia, and had eaten armadillo, which I enjoyed. When I told him about it, he proceeded to expound on armadillos in general – the difference between the three- and six-banded Bolivian armadillos. Of course, I had not thought to ask my hosts to count the number of bands on the animals before cooking them.

But his major problem was his difficulty in communication and, perhaps as a consequence, his poor interpersonal skills. He normally communicated in WHO in English but had studied in France, and his detractors would say that his communication was equally poor in English, French and Japanese, which was his native tongue. Strange as it may seem now, he was protective of WHO and resisted attempts to bypass it. One of his most public disagreements was with Jonathan Mann, a competent, charismatic epidemiologist who was head of the HIV programme. Jonathan's perceptive, expansive vision of an HIV programme did not fit with Dr Nakajima's conservative, cautious approach. This led to Jonathan's public resignation and, in my judgement, was the beginning of the decision to establish the Joint United Nations Programme on HIV/AIDS (UNAIDS) initially as a coordinating agency with WHO as only one participant.

In addition, there was considerable dissatisfaction among the staff, in part because of some poor human resources practices and also because of Dr Nakajima's failure to project a coherent vision and persuade or convince staff to buy into it. This led to several unsavoury rumours and comments on his personal attributes and dealings. It was suggested that some of the opposition was related to political tensions between Japan and the Western countries, but I have discounted this, as there was almost universal admiration for Sadako Ogata in her role as the UN High Commissioner for Refugees from 1991 to 2000.

There was persistent clamour for reform in WHO – a cry that goes on even today, which makes one wonder whether there is clarity about the type of organization that is needed or, rather, that the member states wish. In spite of the numerous conferences about and criticisms of WHO, it was never clear precisely what objectives the proposed reforms would achieve. But there were perhaps a few common threads. First was a call for better leadership. There were calls for greater efficiency, with some governments calling for WHO on the one hand to limit its scope of action and some on the other calling for an expansion into new areas as they arose. But there was one aspect on which there seemed to be consensus – they all wished to reduce their quota contributions to WHO or at least not have them increase. The consequences of the Helms/Biden legislation in the US Senate, which condemned UN agencies from 2001 to zero-negative budget growth, has been a veritable millstone around WHO's neck. This draconian legislation followed the agreement to pay the United States arrears to the United Nations. Little attention was paid to the several accomplishments in international health while Dr Nakajima was director general. When asked my opinion about Dr Nakajima during my campaign, my response was that history would treat him kindly – and I am still of that view.

MY ELECTION CAMPAIGN

In early 1996, there was increasing speculation on whether Dr Nakajima would seek a third term and who might be his successor. In January the executive board of WHO established the criteria for the qualifications and competencies of the new director general. During the early part of that year, several of the governments of the Americas asked my interest in being a candidate, but I always demurred, stating that my primary concern was with the Pan American Health Organization, and in any case, any decision would turn around whether Dr Nakajima would run again, as I would not oppose him. As a matter of principle, I thought that a regional director should not oppose the director general. During the PAHO Directing Council in September, there was considerable discussion of the issue, but Dr Nakajima gave no indication of his intention during his many formal and informal interactions with the health ministers of the Americas.

After the meeting of the executive board of January 1997, the feeling was that Japan was ambivalent and did not wish to see Dr Nakajima pushed out, although the major countries, the United States, the United Kingdom, Canada, made it abundantly clear that they were adamantly opposed to a third term. There was discussion among the Western European countries, the United States, Canada and Australia about a possible candidate, and several of these governments approached Dr Gro Harlem Brundtland, ex-prime minister of Norway, to persuade her to be a candidate. I met with

A New International Challenge: The Director General of the WHO

Dr Nakajima in March and asked him about his intentions, but he would not give a direct answer. I then discussed the matter with our Ministry of Foreign Affairs, which was cautiously enthusiastic about proposing me as a candidate. They wrote formally to the Japanese ambassador in Port of Spain seeking clarification as "both Sir George Alleyne and the Government of Barbados, out of deep respect for Dr Nakajima are extremely reluctant to let Sir George's name go forward if it is known that Dr Nakajima will be seeking another term".

The thinking among the diplomats in Geneva was that Dr Nakajima was considering another term and that the only candidate who would force his hand was Dr Brundtland, and there was a growing feeling that all the other countries, including Barbados, should line up behind her as an ideal candidate. The Barbados Ministry of Foreign Affairs – specifically the minister, Dame Billie Miller, and the permanent secretary, Dr Peter Laurie, contrary to what appeared to be a genuflection to Dr Brundtland, took a completely different approach. They carried out a careful political analysis and decided that Dr Brundtland as a candidate would perhaps force Dr Nakajima's hand, but once he stepped down, Dr Brundtland's position would be completely different, and there were enough positives for my candidature to make it worth the effort.

On 18 March, the Government of Barbados consulted me about a decision to prefer my candidature, and on 4 April, I formally agreed. The analysis by the Ministry of Foreign Affairs was that I fitted perfectly the criteria established by the executive board, and the recognized managerial competence I had displayed at PAHO was what was needed to reform WHO. Their appreciation was that the major issues to be highlighted at WHO were essentially managerial, and there was nothing wrong basically with its capacity to discharge technical, normative functions.

Dr Nakajima formally declared on 29 April that he was not seeking another term, and on 7 May, at the World Health Assembly, Ms Liz Thompson, the minister of health of Barbados, formally announced in her speech to the assembly that Barbados was putting forward Sir George Alleyne as a candidate for the post of director general. I have to confess that my heart skipped several beats as I sat in the hall and heard her make the announcement and outline the rationale for it. Over the course of the next month, it became clear that there were essentially seven serious candidates: Dr Gro Brundtland from Norway; Dr Ebrahim Samba from Zambia, regional director of the WHO African Region; Dr Uton Muchtar Rafei from Indonesia, regional director of WHO South East-Asia Region; Dr Nafis Sadik of Pakistan, executive director of United Nations Population Fund; Dr Fernando Antezana from Bolivia and currently deputy director of WHO and myself.

One analysis in the Ministry of Foreign Affairs concluded that the strongest candidates were Dr Brundtland, Dr Sadik and myself. A strategic plan was designed involving every one of Barbados' diplomatic missions as well as incorporating all of CARICOM. The CARICOM Heads of Governments formally endorsed the candidature at their meeting in June 1997, and I recall a moment of comedy during this process. Owen Arthur, prime minister of Barbados, presented my candidature, explained the reason why Barbados was optimistic, stressed the need for CARICOM solidarity and support, and asked for comments. Every one of the heads of government gave enthusiastic support, but Jamaica demurred, and the prime minister of Jamaica, P.J. Patterson, said something like this: "Colleagues, I understand the enthusiasm of Barbados – I know the candidate and his qualifications very well, but he has a serious flaw which he cannot correct." There was dead silence. Then Prime Minister Patterson went on. "He was in the wrong Hall." At which there was loud laughter, especially since the majority of the prime ministers were alumni of the University of the West Indies. Mr Patterson was alluding to the fact that he and I were students together at the University College of the West Indies at Mona, and I was in Taylor Hall while he was in Chancellor Hall, between which there was and has always been intense rivalry.

There was intensive lobbying at the World Health Assembly in May 1997, as Norway had a delegation of about thirty persons, and it appeared that they were everywhere at every event, buttonholing the various delegates and pressing Dr Brundtland's case. The Barbados delegation was three – the minister, the permanent secretary, and the chief medical officer. Peter Simmons, the high commissioner in London, came to Geneva for the post World Health Assembly meeting of the executive board and engaged in intensive lobbying, especially among his colleague diplomats, and as a

A New International Challenge: The Director General of the WHO

result advised the ministry that the climate was propitious, and it should be more aggressive as there was general recognition of the competence of its candidate and the extent to which he satisfied perfectly the criteria that had been established. Dr Brundtland asked to see me during the assembly, and I met her in an office that had been assigned to her. This was the first time I was meeting her, and I was impressed by her directness. We exchanged pleasantries, and she explained briefly that she thought she would make a good director general; I did the same. We simply took measure of each other, agreed that there would be no negative campaigning and wished each other good luck.

There was a comical incident during the assembly, when I met with Dr Sadik, at her request, to discuss our chances. She was very positive, to put it mildly, and at the end said something like this: "George, I will win. I have an advantage over you in that I am a woman." To which I replied, "Well, that is something I cannot change." When I recounted the incident to David Dingwall, former minister of health of Canada, who was supporting me, I repeated her comment that she was a woman. He enquired as to my response, and when I told him that I had responded by saying that I could not change that, quick as a flash, he said, "No, George, that was the wrong response. When she said that she had an advantage because she was a woman, you should have replied, 'How do you know I am not?'"

The intelligence gained from the World Health Assembly was all collated with that from the diplomatic missions of Barbados and of CARICOM countries, and on 28 May 1997, the Ministry of Foreign Affairs again revised the strategy. The assessment was that Dr Brundtland was indeed the leading candidate – she was a former prime minister, well known internationally, and the announcement of her availability under pressure from the United States, United Kingdom, Canada and Australia was a contributing factor to Dr Nakajima's decision. She would probably have had the support of the European countries, but there was a suspicion that her declared "availability" was because she was still interested in being secretary general of the United Nations. She put that speculation to rest in an open letter declaring that WHO was her single focus. The point was made again that given the interest of the executive board in WHO reform and its efficient management and my demonstrated managerial competence in PAHO, my candidature was seen positively by enough countries to warrant an aggressive campaign. One of the keys to success was in securing the support of some of the major contributors to WHO, especially those who were members of the executive board. So the first objective of the campaign was to convince those major countries that I was the person with the managerial skills who could best achieve the goals they had established, since all wished to establish sound management in WHO.

This strategy set out in minute and impressive detail the roles of the various offices, the message they should convey, and the form and periodicity of the communications. It set out the situation of every one of the executive board countries, what was their voting record in various international fora, who should approach them, the lobbying points that might best convince them, and the action to be taken by the various individuals, mainly West Indians who were likely to be helpful. It was noted that I was the second choice of the United States, United Kingdom and Canada, all of whom had approached Dr Brundtland to run.

The most significant event of the summer of 1997 was the decision of Canada to support me. I found out that this was due to the influence of David Dingwall, whom I had met and with whom I had had long conversations on several occasions previously in PAHO. Canada had indeed approached Dr Brundtland to run, but Mr Dingwall convinced Prime Minister Chrétien that it was in Canada's interest to support a Caribbean candidate and that this support should be active rather than passive. I gather that Canada's decision was not well received in Norway!

The Ministry of Foreign Affairs decided that a presentation brochure was needed, and a public relations firm, Ruder Finn, was contracted to develop a media communication strategy and to assist in the preparation of the brochure. This received positive comments universally, and the fact that it was in all the official WHO languages as well as Korean was a plus. I was fortunate to have been able to incorporate the comments I received from my predecessor and several international health experts who were my friends, such as Dr Adetokunbo Lucas and Dr Julio Frenk.

I attended the Commonwealth Heads of Government meeting in Edinburgh in October 1997 and made a presentation to several of the ministers of foreign affairs or their deputies. Prime Minister Arthur was

A New International Challenge: The Director General of the WHO

complimentary, saying that it was now crystal clear to him why I wished to be director general and what I proposed to do when I was elected. All the participants were complimentary and I believe impressed, but several, such as Australia, had already committed to supporting Dr Brundtland. By then I had made visits to Peru, Brazil, Canada, Egypt, United Kingdom, Japan, Argentina, Germany, Croatia, Holland, Bahrain and the United Arab Emirates. I was well received in all the countries, and some, such as Argentina, Bahrain and Egypt, were open in declaring their support for me. I had also visited Geneva and interviewed representatives of every one of the executive board members and had even included a visit to the Papal Nuncio there. Of course we lobbied the United States through the State Department and Dr Donna Shalala, secretary for health and human services of the United States, kindly invited me to lunch. She was non-committal but did emphasize that I was a good candidate and that there should be no negative campaigning.

In our several strategy sessions in the Ministry of Foreign Affairs, there was constant comment on the importance of the African vote, and several contacts were made at various levels in those countries – Angola, Burundi, Benin, Botswana, Zimbabwe, Burkino Faso and Algeria. I even called and spoke to Julius Nyerere, the former president of Tanzania, myself. He was unhelpful and spoke to me of the support Tanzania had received from Norway and of Dr Brundtland's international profile. Our consensus was that it was not profitable to visit these countries, as the experience was that commitments made at senior levels were not always honoured, and in addition there seemed to be agreement that as a group they would support Samba on the first ballot. But in large part due to Cuban intervention, there was a formal support from Angola at least on the second ballot.

So Sylvan and I went off to Geneva for the decisive meeting of the executive board in January 1998, where the voting would take place. The Barbados delegation to the executive board comprised minister of foreign affairs Dame Billie Miller, minister of health Liz Thompson, permanent secretary Dr Peter Laurie, chief medical officer Dr Elizabeth Ferdinand, ambassadors in London, Geneva and Brussels, and Branford Taitt. Mr Taitt's addition to the delegation was interesting. He was then a member of the opposition but had been minister of health before and was well recognized and highly regarded in international health circles, so it was felt that he would be of value to the campaign. This was an example of the candidature being one put forward by Barbados as a whole and not by any particular political party.

I have reviewed my handwritten notes made just before leaving for Geneva. I reflected in them on the fact that, in my professional career, I had always been successful in overcoming the challenges put before me and indeed had never lost a major contest. The thought did cross my mind that perhaps the Peter Principle could come into play, and I had at last reached the pinnacle of my competence and would go no further. I also reflected on the sophistication and professional nature of the campaign that Barbados had mounted. Just then I was amused to read an article from the *Economist* about choosing the president of the European Central Bank. It read as follows: "Any senior international job offers an excuse for political horse-trading. The spectacle of governments exerting political muscle, calling in old favors or trading off new ones may be unedifying, but it is the time-tested way of international politics and little harm is usually done." So much for talent and competence!

I was comfortable as I approached the meeting of the executive board that everything possible had been done. I had been well coached for my oral presentation by Dr Eve Epstein, who had also coached Kofi Annan. I prided myself on my ability to communicate, but I have to admit that she improved my presentation significantly, and I was grateful to her for it. But just before leaving for Geneva, Dr Donna Shalala called to tell me that her government, although it would not be on the executive board and therefore would not be voting, would be favouring Gro Brundtland, but they recognized my qualifications and would not be lobbying against me. This was not the unkindest cut of all, but fairly close, but I philosophized that the United States was one of the countries that had approached Dr Brundtland initially and perhaps felt that it had to honour that commitment. Also, I had to recognize that as Otto Abbadabba, the Mafia accountant, said famously and undoubtedly in relation to the disappearance of some rival, "It was nothing personal it was just business."

I had prepared a special document in English and French on my ideas on the health problems in Africa and how WHO should address them, and I

A New International Challenge: The Director General of the WHO

presented it to the African members of the executive board and other African missions in Geneva during the week of the executive board meetings. Interestingly, many of them were enthusiastic about supporting me and all wished me good luck.

A most unpleasant incident occurred, however, during that week before the voting took place. One of the representatives from an African country approached me directly and asked for money for his vote and that of another colleague. I was both annoyed and embarrassed at the effrontery – by the fact that he thought he could approach me, and I was embarrassed to have proof positive of the corruption that occurs in these processes. I informed him as firmly as I could that Barbados did not buy votes. Our analysis of the voting pattern afterwards indicated to us quite clearly where his votes and those of his colleague were cast. Perhaps I should be charitable and believe that this was an isolated incident by a disreputable representative. That convinced me that the system was broken. I had no doubt that he had his instructions from his government, but because there is secret balloting, he could seek to flog his vote. I was then even more persuaded that the system will continue to be open to corruption until there is open voting, which will make it clear how every country has voted.

Our campaign had noted with chagrin that Commonwealth ties had no relevance, and it was doubtful that developing-world solidarity would play any role, especially since four of the candidates were from that part of the world. But in a last ditch effort to achieve some kind of consensus, Dr Ismail Sallam, minister of health of Egypt invited Mr Taitt and myself to a dinner at the home of the Egyptian ambassador along with Dr Samba, Dr Sadik and representatives from Dr Uton's team. Dr Sallam put it bluntly: any dispassionate analysis of the candidates showed that I was likely to gain majority support, and if the others agreed to support me, I would win. He pleaded for support at least on the second ballot. Mr Taitt was brilliant in his presentation of the history of developing world fragmentation and the persistent dreams and rhetoric of solidarity. He dilated on the need to demonstrate developing world capabilities and its capacity for mutual trust and collective action. This was to no avail. Dr Samba spoke but said nothing; Dr Sadik was clear that as a woman, she had the best chance of winning against Dr Brundtland; and Dr Uton's representatives offered a bilateral agreement with Barbados if it would commit to him being deputy director general – which of course was not possible, as I have always been of the view that the organization's positions were not to be decided in that manner. Thus there was no decision, and as Dr Sallam would say ruefully, "I tried."

THE ELECTION

As the day dawned on the morning of my presentation, Sylvan awoke me and told me that she was concerned as she had just heard a cock crow thrice, which of course for Christians is significant, as it evokes the betrayal of Jesus in the garden of Gethsemane. I did not take the symbolism or augury as seriously as she did.

I made my presentation at 2:30 p.m. on 25 January. I did not use slides and spoke for thirty minutes without notes. I elaborated on the problems of the organization, the kinds of reform that it needed, as well as the managerial skills and tools that should be applied and which I possessed. I cast health as one of the instruments of human development and emphasized that a health organization should play a role as an instrument of that development. I touched on the need for a lofty vision, a practical mission and the ways they should be achieved. I referred to the need for equity and social justice and pointed out that any process of reform must begin with an appreciation of our value system, which should include service, equity, international solidarity and technical excellence. I pointed out the need for an organizational structure to reflect my philosophy, with which I hoped they agreed, but I mentioned some specific programme areas which would need special attention and emphasized the need for support to Africa. I ended by citing the five major principles that would guide the reform. These would be adumbration of the core values, strengthening WHO as a centre of excellence in health, streamlining the secretariat, ensuring fiscal and programmatic transparency and emphasizing partnerships. In my peroration, I encouraged the members to share with me my vision of a reformed WHO and a concept of health that was for me a magnificent obsession.

I answered concisely the various questions put to me and was pleased to be able to respond to the delegate from Argentina in Spanish. By all

A New International Challenge: The Director General of the WHO

accounts my presentation was excellent, and I am told that some members of the Barbados dedication wept with pride. More than one member government congratulated me on my presentation, and at least two said ruefully, "But I have my instructions." In a letter to me subsequently, the editor of the *Lancet* described my presentation as an "honest, welcome and humble criticism that must have been very difficult for the Executive Board to resist".

I then retired to my office to sit quietly with Sylvan and await the results of the ballot, which went to four rounds, and then Peter Laurie came to tell me of the result. Dr Brundtland had won. We listened to her acceptance speech, and then I came from my office to meet and greet her. I congratulated her and offered her my full support. She accepted graciously and suggested that we should meet the next time she was in Washington.

We carried out the best analysis we could of what we imagined was the voting pattern, and it was clear to us that the European countries remained with Dr Brundtland solidly throughout, and over the course of the ballots she gained support from other regions. Our analysis was that except for Angola, no African country voted for me.

In retrospect I was amazingly calm about the result, in large part due to Sylvan's presence. This was the first time I had lost any contest. This was the first time I had wished to be preeminent, and the laurel was denied me. During the next forty-eight hours I kept repeating to myself the famous lines from Kipling: "If you can meet with Triumph and Disaster / and treat those imposters just the same . . ."

I have had many triumphs in life, and reflection and Sylvan's comforting words made me see quickly that the result of the election should not be seen as a disaster. I could receive that night with equanimity and much pleasure a telephone call from the prime minister of Barbados, who told me how proud he and the country were of the way our campaign had been run and how I had performed. He too did not see it as a disaster. One of my overriding thoughts was gratitude to the people of Barbados, especially the prime minister, the staff of the Ministry of Foreign Affairs, especially the minister herself, Dame Billie Miller, Permanent Secretary Dr Peter Laurie, and the Ministry of Health led by Ms Liz Thompson, for the tremendous effort they put into the campaign. I was impressed by the capacity of a small country like ours to mount such an organized global effort that was everywhere recognized as being professional and brilliantly executed. I also know that it was not cheap, but I do hope they think it was worth it. I must also mention the support from the other CARICOM countries, which were enthusiastic about the campaign.

I received numerous letters, cards and telephone calls of congratulations from many parts of the world and was especially touched by the champagne reception given by my staff the day I returned to PAHO. But perhaps the nicest comment of all was made by my six-year-old grandson, who said to me, "Grandpa, I am sorry you lost the election, but I'm glad that you are not going anywhere."

Three months later, the prime minister wrote me this letter:

> Dear Sir George,
>
> It is incumbent on me let you know how proud my Government and the people of Barbados are of the exemplary manner in which you represented Barbados and the region in the election for the post of Director General of the World Health Organization.
>
> It is indeed unfortunate that despite our best efforts and the acknowledgement that you were the ideal candidate, you were unable to secure the coveted position. You and the Barbadian delegation must however be complimented for having run a dignified campaign which will redound to the credit and character of the Barbadian personality.
>
> I wish to commend you for your outstanding performance and assure you of my Government's continued support for your efforts in the international health arena.
>
> Yours sincerely,
> Owen S. Arthur
> Prime Minister

CHAPTER 10

A Second Term as Director

I engaged in considerable soul searching as to what I should do next. Should I retire gracefully from international life or seek a second term as director of PAHO? I was now sixty-six years old, but I still retained considerable enthusiasm for my work and felt that there was still much to be done to push forward the notions of equity and pan-Americanism. Of course, such is the nature of these organizations that there was no shortage of persons encouraging me to seek a second term.

James Collins is one of the authors of a popular book on management entitled *Built to Last: The Successful Habits of Visionary Companies*,[1] which repeats the nostrums of books of a similar genre and establishes the so-called secrets of business success. I enjoyed reading them and their prescriptions, but one of Collins's ideas struck me forcibly. He wrote of BHAGs – big, hairy, audacious goals – which he advocated as powerful mechanisms to stimulate progress. I thought of it in terms of PAHO and of me as director in particular.

These thoughts were very much in my mind when I was re-elected unopposed in 1998. In my presentation to the Sanitary Conference, I recalled:

> those occasions on which we have witnessed together simple activities in the places in which your people, my people, live and love and labour and die. I will always recall the tiny tots of the Tacuarembó in Uruguay; the proud people of Pocri in Panama; the women of Chiclayo in Peru, who soldered silos to protect their harvest grains from rats that brought them the plague; the Tenement Yard in Trench Town, Jamaica, where Bob Marley cooked his

cornmeal porridge. I could go on and on. These were the places in which I could hear and see and feel the various ways health was being improved and our organization is proud to be a part of your efforts.

Enrique Iglesias, president of the Inter-American Development Bank, invited me and the ministers to lunch at the bank that day, and there I declared that for the next four years I would have two personal BHAGs. The first would be to fashion an agenda for health in the Americas that would have the active involvement of the World Bank and the Inter-American Development Bank. The second was to revisit public health practice in a fundamental way, articulating the essential functions to be carried out that fell within the regulatory or steering role of the public health sector of government. I envisaged a centennial publication that would establish the functions that the state should discharge if the public's health was to be promoted and avoidable illness prevented.

The three agencies developed and signed formally a "Shared Agenda for Health in the Americas", which was based on shared institutional objectives:

- to contribute effectively to improve the health of the peoples of the Americas through activities in environment, disease prevention and control, and strengthening of the health services;
- to reduce, and eliminate, to the extent possible, avoidable inequalities in health conditions and in access to health services and basic sanitation;
- to institutionally strengthen and improve the efficacy, efficiency, and effectiveness of the services of the public and private health systems; and
- to encourage greater synergy between health and social and economic development, using – among other means – evaluations of the health impact of programmes on different aspects of development

This achieved modest success but lapsed when the president of the Inter-American Development Bank, the responsible vice president of the World Bank, and I demitted office.

The work on the second was ably led by Daniel Lopez Acuna, director of the Division of Health Systems and Services Development, and involved many actors within and outside of PAHO. There was much discussion and debate about the renewal of public health and the concepts and practice that should obtain. Eventually eleven essential public health functions were established and ratified by the member states:

1. monitoring, evaluation, and analysis of health status
2. public health surveillance, research and control of risks and threats to public health
3. health promotion
4. social participation in health
5. development of policies and institutional capacity for planning and management in public health
6. strengthening of institutional capacity for regulation and enforcement in public health
7. evaluation and promotion of equitable access to the necessary health services
8. human resources development and training in public health
9. quality assurance in personal and population-based health services
10. research in public health
11. reduction of the impact of emergencies and disasters on health

Note that all of these cannot be the unique responsibility of the Ministry of Health. They require whole-of-government as well as whole-of-society approaches, and neither is easily accomplished. Although there was emphasis on essential public health functions, these were part of the broader initiative "Public Health in the Americas",[2] which had the following main objectives: development of a regional definition of the essential public health functions; development of instruments to measure their performance as the basis for improving public health practice; and development of the methodology and instruments to support the formulation and implementation of some national, subregional and regional lines of action that will help to strengthen the public health infrastructure and thereby enhance the leadership of the health authority at all levels of the state.

There had been considerable discussion and debate on current public health practice in the recent past. In collaboration with the Association of Schools of Public Health of the United States and the Latin American and Caribbean Association for Education in Public Health, PAHO had embarked in 1988 on an ambitious programme to redefine public health practice and teaching, especially in relation to the goal of Health for All by the Year 2000. There had been an impressive publication "The Crisis of Public Health: Reflection for the Debate",[3] which had examined the very conceptual basis of public health and had even postulated a new public health whose essential focus was at the population level, drawing a clear separation of that discipline from the practice of clinical medicine.

I have always been reluctant about developing new theories or practices and have preferred to build upon or certainly make reference to established precepts. I believed that the concept of public health as "the science and art of preventing disease, prolonging life and promoting health through the organized efforts of society" remained valid. It had become clearer that the society of reference involved all three parts of the state – governments, private sector and civil society – although the major responsibility lay with the government that had at its disposal the key regulatory instruments.

I am pleased that the concept of essential public health functions, although lying dormant for some time, is being resuscitated and that at least one other regional office has developed its own set of essential public health functions and the tools necessary to measure if these are being carried out to strengthen public health practice.

THE WORK OF PAHO

It is impossible to give details of the work of PAHO over the eight years in which I was director, but summaries can be found in my annual reports, and the work during my second term is outlined in my final quadrennial report, a richly illustrated document which celebrates many of the more significant achievements. Our technical cooperation was carried out with a staff of just over two thousand, two-thirds of whom were at the country level. The budget for our final biennium was approximately US$375 million, the majority of which came from the contributions of the countries and eighty-five per cent was spent on regional and country programmes. The major technical areas in which we worked and which were reflected in the organizational structure were Health and Human Development, Disease Prevention and Control, Health Promotion and Protection,

A Second Term as Director

Environmental Health and Protection, and Health Systems and Services. PAHO also administered five regional centres. I will highlight a few of the accomplishments.

The Division of Health and Human Development included our Research and Bioethics programmes and was responsible for our work on the relationship between health and other dimensions of human development, particularly economic growth. This had been a particular area of interest of mine for the previous twenty-odd years. We initiated work on the nexus among health, development and tourism, which is of special ongoing interest to the Caribbean.

We devoted considerable attention to getting core data on health and made considerable progress in spreading the practice of epidemiology and health situation analysis at the country level and using tools such as geospatial mapping. We were pleased to see the practice of developing and publishing core health data sets used in other WHO regions.

The programme of Women, Health and Development was special, as I had recognized early that many of the problems of the health of women were rooted not in their biology but in pernicious and pervasive gender discrimination. There had been a committee on women, health and development and a small programme with one professional staff member, but I established a larger formal technical programme to provide cooperation to our member countries in the subject area. The concept of gender and how it impacted on health was not well understood in our region. The popular perception was that it was related primarily to the place of women in society and particularly in the workplace.

I would often recount the story of my visit to a rural clinic in one of our countries and being told of a woman who had died of pre-partum haemorrhage. She began to bleed but could not go to the hospital for attention until her husband came home to give permission and take her. By that time, it was too late. This is an extreme but not isolated example of male domination. I was often asked why I resisted changing the title of the programme to the more fashionable and perhaps more appropriate "Gender and Development". My obstinate reply was that I would agree to the change in name when I could be persuaded that men were equally discriminated against. Much of my concern for the gender dimension of health was captured in a lecture I gave much later entitled "Health Degendered Is Health Denied". As another indication of my commitment to increasing gender equity, I continued the practice of including a strong appeal for governments to include more women in their delegations attending the meetings of the PAHO governing bodies.

The tradition of excellence in disease prevention and control continued. The programme on immunization led the world. As I mentioned before, the region of the Americas was the first to eliminate poliomyelitis and measles, in no small measure due to the charisma and drive of the head of the programme, Ciro de Quadros, who was ably supported by a dedicated, committed group of professionals whom he inspired and sometimes drove with almost messianic zeal. We were well on the way to eliminating the mother-to-child transmission of HIV. HIV/AIDS was a major challenge, and progress was slow in large part due to the prohibitive cost of drugs. PAHO was proud of the veterinary public health programme and the work in food safety. The programme on the eradication of foot-and-mouth disease was outstanding, and the success was due in great part to the work of our Pan American Center for Foot and Mouth Disease, whose epidemiological surveillance of the disease was the envy of human health.

The Division of Health Promotion and Protection encompassed the traditional maternal and child health programmes, which saw a steady decline in maternal and child mortality throughout the region. The mental health programme introduced innovations such as the training of hairdressers to recognize early depression, and there were advances in linking mental health to human rights and alleviating the horrible conditions of custodial care.

The Division of Environmental Health and Protection devoted considerable attention to improving the regional water supply and sanitation systems. The elimination of lead from gasoline in the region is an achievement of which we were proud. Because of the frequency of natural disasters in the Americas, PAHO had established a technical programme in disaster preparedness, which succeeded in strengthening hemispheric cooperation and national capacities to develop an integrated approach to the management of natural disasters. Its training materials were used as far afield as Japan.

A Second Term as Director

We always recognized that strengthening health systems was the bedrock of service provision for all sections of the population. The technical cooperation therefore focused on the essential components of the health system, especially human resources management and health financing, which occupied most attention in the programmes of health sector reform which the countries embraced. We supported countries in their difficult task of measuring health system performance. Other areas of technical cooperation included oral health, in which promotion of salt fluoridation lead to significant decrease in dental caries, health services engineering, and supporting laboratory and blood services, the latter making significant progress in promoting voluntary blood donation.

Our publications programme was outstanding. PAHO's website was introduced, and we launched several programmes of public information to sensitize the public on our work. We collaborated with a wide range of partners, and an honour roll of partners (never donors) included other governments, international organizations, private and public sector organizations and even faith-based organizations.

Among PAHO's strengths is its convening power: its response to emergencies and the ability to secure cooperation with other UN agencies. One example was in the control of cholera in Central America. In 1991, after an absence of nearly a century, cholera appeared in Peru and in the first two years affected fourteen countries, causing about one million cases with about nine thousand deaths. The basic cause was a poor sanitary infrastructure, especially in relation to water. The epidemic was brought under control, but then in 1998, Hurricane Mitch, the deadliest Atlantic hurricane in two hundred years, provoked widespread devastation in Central America, causing more than eleven thousand deaths and a rebound of the cholera epidemic.

I met with the ministers of health of Central America in Costa del Sol in El Salvador and signed a formal agreement which stipulated that PAHO would coordinate an ambitious plan for investment in health and the environment. They accepted my offer of one million dollars to begin putting the plan into effect. A few days later, I met with Carol Bellamy, the executive director of UNICEF, and asked her to cooperate with us. She agreed and on the spot pledged half a million US dollars. PAHO and UNICEF worked together in a joint effort which happily saw the epidemic brought under control in four years. I often cite this as an example of PAHO's capacity for immediate response to a crisis situation and the trust reposed in us by other agencies to work cooperatively at country level. It also demonstrated how carefully planned and adequately financed public health interventions can have measurable outcomes.

The political dimension was never ignored, and I participated in the Hemispheric Summits of the Americas in 1994, 1998 and 2001, in which I had the opportunity to address the political leaders of the Americas. The 1998 summit had raised the awareness of the importance of health to human rights and poverty alleviation, and I participated in a roundtable with Hillary Clinton, then First Lady of the United States, on the importance of health to the preservation of democracy. I also welcomed the opportunity to participate in and host meetings of the First Ladies of the Americas who were critical allies in the domestic promotion of our programmes.

I am particularly pleased and proud of my relationship with our member governments. During my term of office, I met at one time or another with every one of the presidents or prime ministers of the Americas. They showed varying degrees of interest in health, and perhaps the one who was most deeply interested and personally involved was Fidel Castro, president of Cuba. He took a keen, personal interest in all aspects of health, both of his country and of the world as a whole, and was quite appropriately immensely proud of the advances Cuba had made in all aspects of health. In long fascinating conversations with me, sometimes at odd hours in the night, he would elaborate on why health was such a critical aspect of Cuba's development. Cuba's health indicators were among the best in the world, in spite of the country's economic problems. He paid particular attention to the development of biotechnology, and the national centre, which, to the surprise of many international visitors, was one of, if not the finest in Latin America.

These visits to the countries were critical to maintaining support for and trust in the organization as well as strengthening the position of the local representative and the office. I continued the practice of inviting new ministers of health to Washington, giving them the opportunity to present

A Second Term as Director

their programmes and interact with the headquarters staff. The mutual respect between us contributed in no small measure to the efficient manner in which the business of the organization was conducted, especially in our governing bodies.

My relations with WHO were in general cordial. I respected Dr Brundtland's position as director general, but that did not stop me on occasion from expressing views that were contrary to those of some of her senior advisers. I admired her courage, for example, in confronting the tobacco industry and getting the countries to agree to a treaty on tobacco control. I had special regard for the competence and professionalism of most of her advisers, but especially for Julio Frenk, a Mexican who was in charge of perhaps the most important division, the one dealing with health systems. She was also well served by her very able senior administrator, Denis Aiken. I think I was sometimes considered a bit of a maverick, but I do not think there was ever animus in our exchanges in the senior staff meetings, and at least when I retired, I was told that my inputs were positive and contributed to the work of the organization.

The year 2002 saw many functions held in my honour and I received several decorations from the governments of the Americas. The CARICOM ministers of health met in a special session in Georgetown, Guyana, which was chaired by Dr Denzil Douglas, prime minister of St Kitts and Nevis. There were several congratulatory speeches, and I was presented with a beautiful album of photographs of some of the special occasions of my life. My emotional reply attempted to show the extent to which, to use the words of Paul to Timothy, "I have fought the good fight, I have finished the race. I have kept the faith."

My focus was more on the last.

NO SADNESS OF FAREWELL

As I demitted office on 30 January 2003, I addressed the staff finally and asked that there be no sadness of farewell on my departure. I reviewed some of the successes and failures of our eight years together. I first paid tribute to my predecessors and said that I and those who came after me as well must recognize that our achievements will be but apostrophes to the names and deeds of my predecessors and the staff who supported them. I recognized the value and virtue of my initial commitment to equity and pan-Americanism and repeated my adherence to the critical value of information in all its forms to the secretariat and our technical cooperation.

As I had said once, "Information is the loom upon which we weave the Pan American shawl that covers and embraces all our countries and facilitates the description and reduction of the inequities in health that must be our constant concern."

I made special mention of our flagship publication *Health in the Americas* and noted the successful initiative of developing the Virtual Health Library of the Americas.

I commented on the many partnerships we had established, particularly with the international financing institutions and several countries outside of the Americas. We had not ignored our hemispheric partners, working closely with the subregional health secretariats, and I was at pains to mention our relationship with CARICOM. I was pleased with our partnerships with WHO over the eight years and believed that we had both learned and taught, but I pointed out that there was still much more to be done to create a unified WHO. I was satisfied with the structural modifications we had made as we had successfully remodelled our headquarters building.

I cited our successful centennial celebrations, at which the United Nations secretary general, Kofi Annan, spoke and honoured our founders and our health heroes and saluted PAHO for the work it had done, was doing and would continue to do. I spoke at length about the trust within the organization and my pride at the degree of it between myself and senior managers, especially those at country level. In my addresses to them over the eight years I had frequently cited the Pygmalion effect, in which I believe strongly. I made no apologies for my emphasis on the need for planning, programming and evaluation in which we had advanced considerably. One of my regrets was that dengue was still rampant in the Americas, because the mosquito Aedes aegypti was to be found in almost every country. This was particularly galling, as one of my predecessors, Fred Soper, had led the countries in the elimination of the mosquito from most of the Americas.

A Second Term as Director

I mentioned some of my personal memories, citing the tears of a cacique of a Bolivian village at seeing clean water coming from a well PAHO had dug. I also recalled with humour the disappointment of the leader of a woman's group in rural Peru when she learned that I was married.

My staff had been tremendous, and I thanked them all for their loyalty, but more importantly, for their support and commitment to the improvement of health in the Americas. I was proud of the simple but elegant vision we had crafted and the extent to which we had realized it.

Our vision was to be the major catalyst for ensuring that all the peoples of the Americas enjoy optimal health and contribute to the well-being of their families and community.

I believed that we had been faithful to that vision.

And so, I left PAHO after twenty-one years.

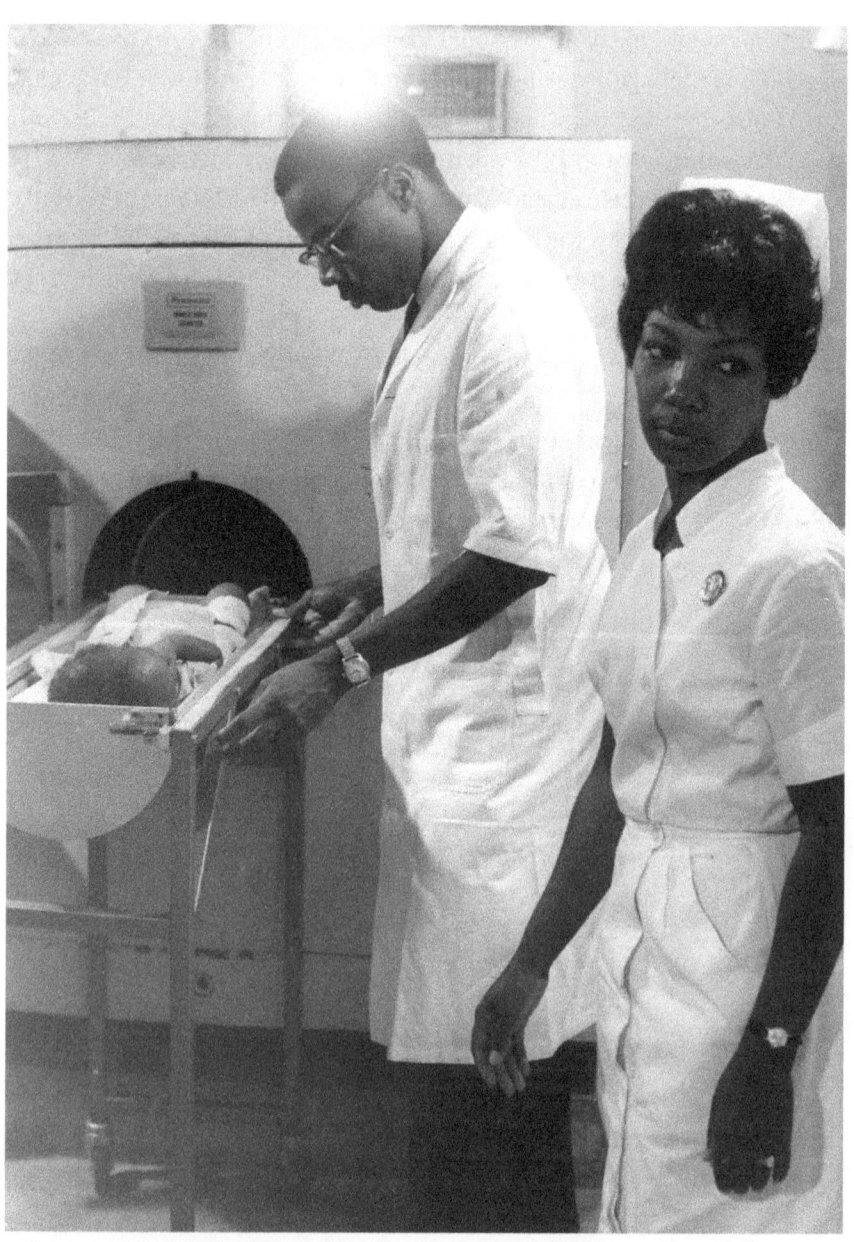

Placing a child in the whole body counter, research in the Tropical Metabolism Research Unit, TMRU around 1968

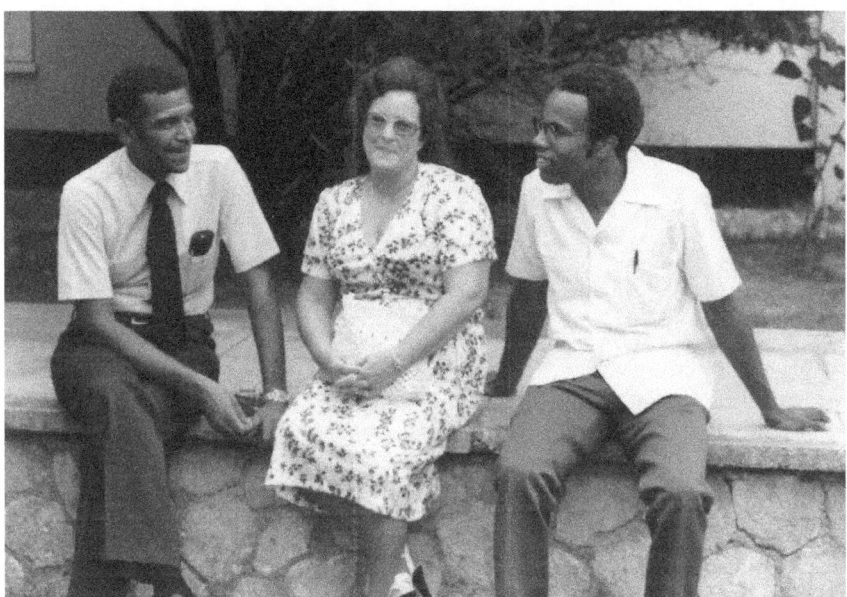

With Professor Hugh Wynter and Noelle Lalor, Department of Medicine, University of the West Indies, Mona

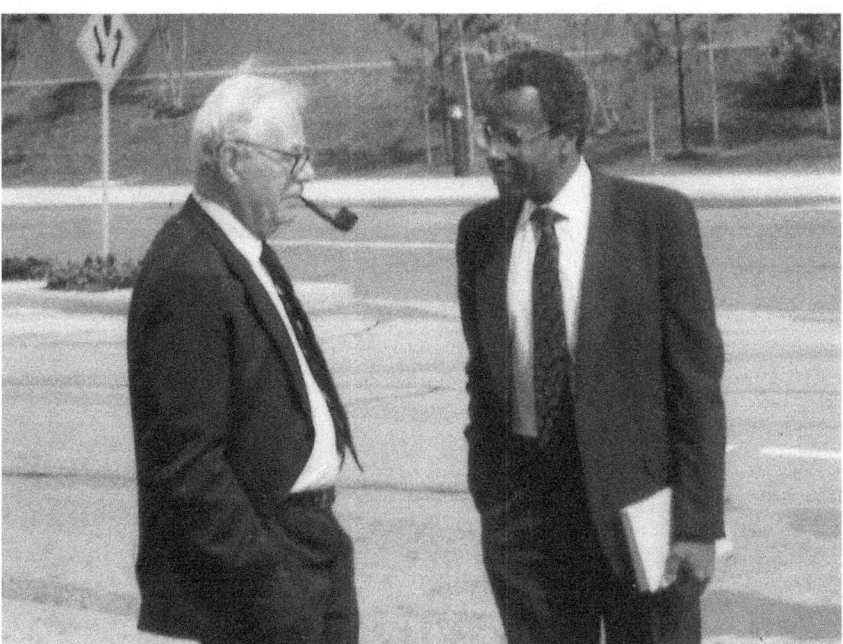

With Professor John Waterlow, Baylor Children's Nutrition Research Center, Texas, 1978

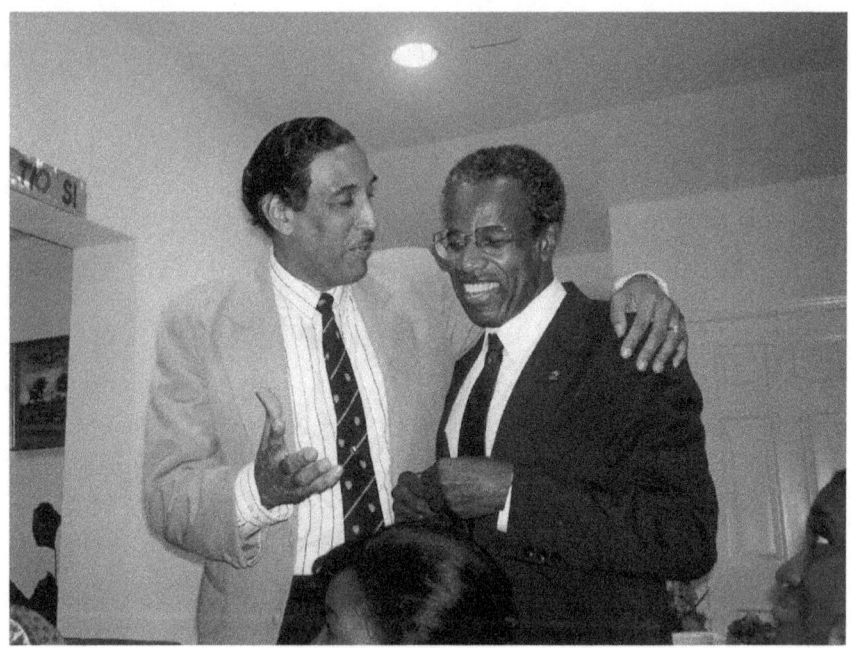

With Knox Hagley, my best friend, 1994

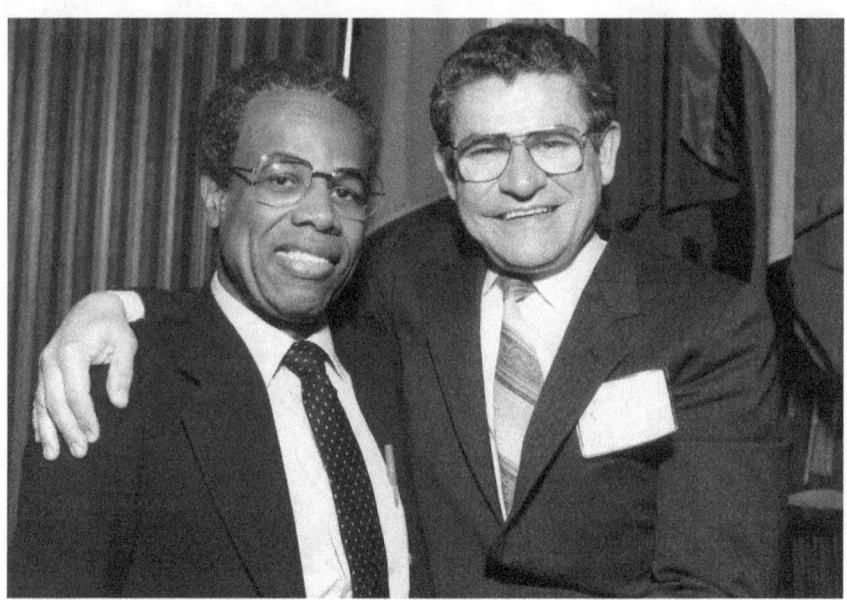

As assistant director of PAHO with Dr Carlyle Guerra de Macedo, director, 1992

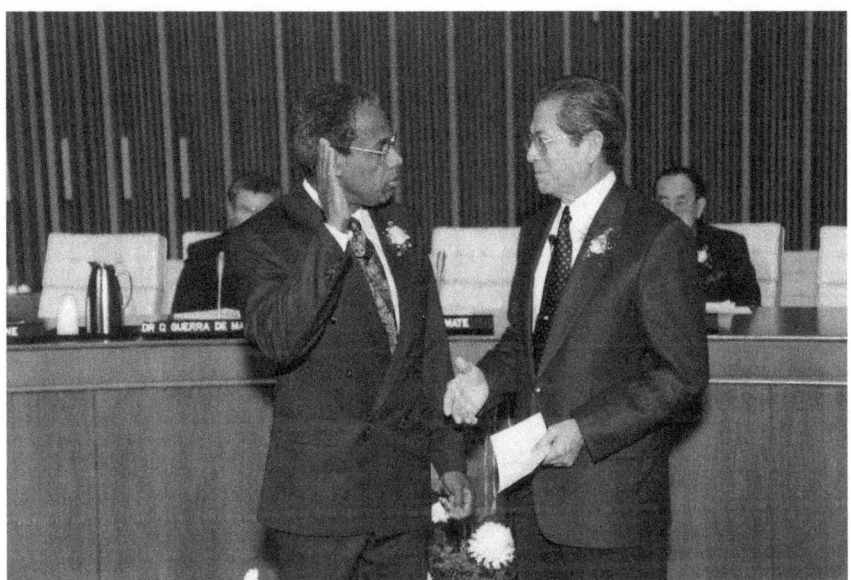

Taking the oath of office as director of PAHO, 31 January 1995, with Dr Jesus Kumate, minister of health of Mexico

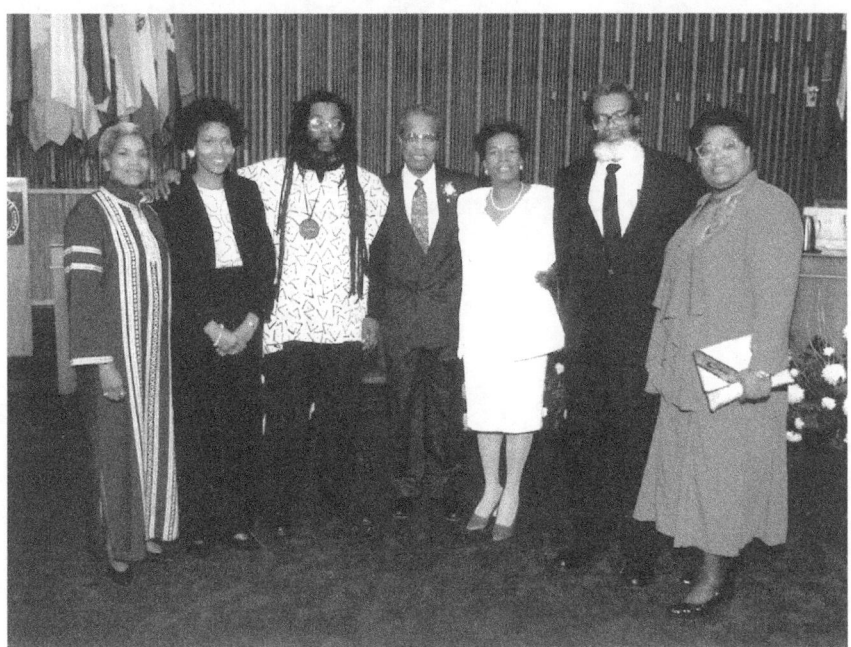

With my six siblings (from left to right), Cynthia, Jacqueline, Peter, Cecily, Grant and Leonora at my installation as director of PAHO, 31 January 1995

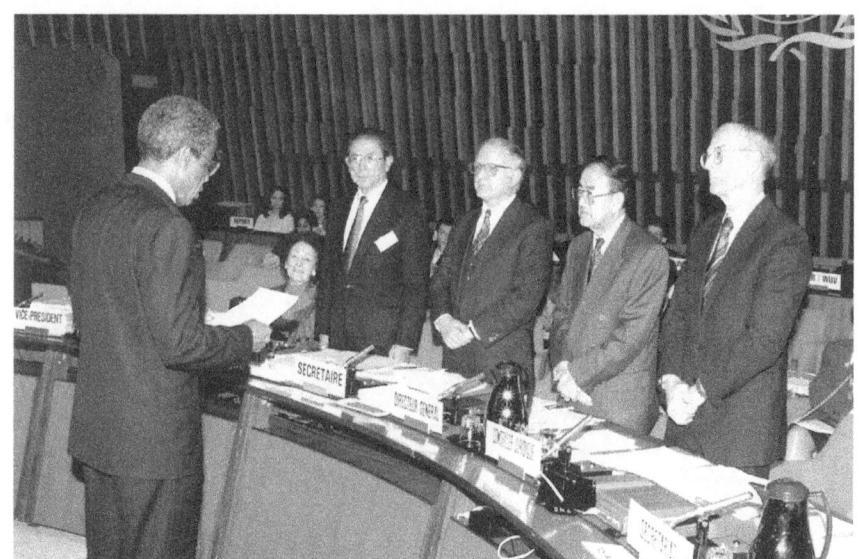

Taking the oath as regional director of WHO for the Americas, January 1995

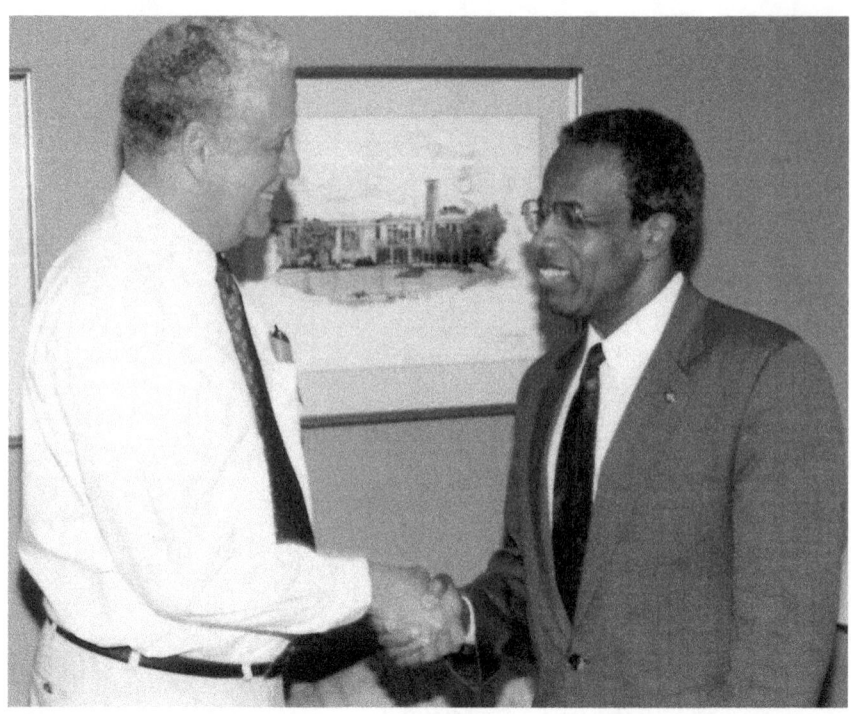

Greeting Vice Chancellor Sir Alister McIntyre at the University of the West Indies, 1995

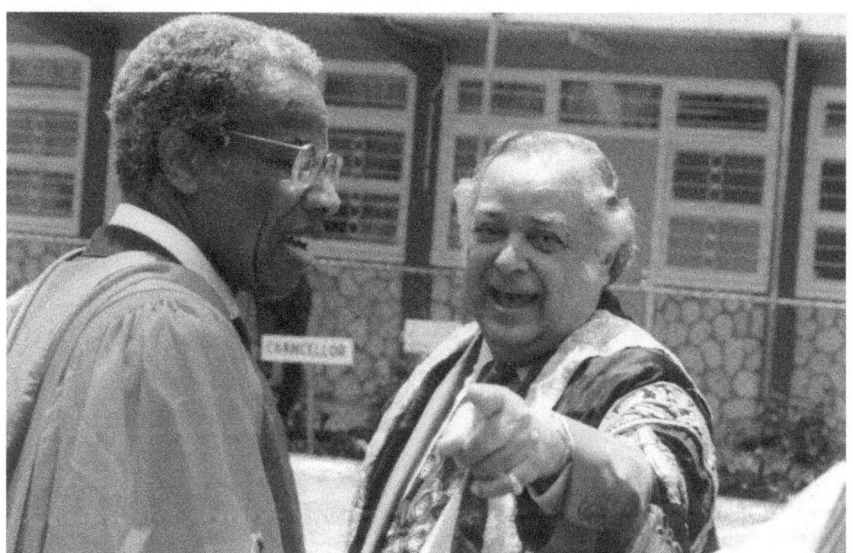

With Chancellor Sir Shridath Ramphal at the fiftieth anniversary celebrations at the University of the West Indies, 1998

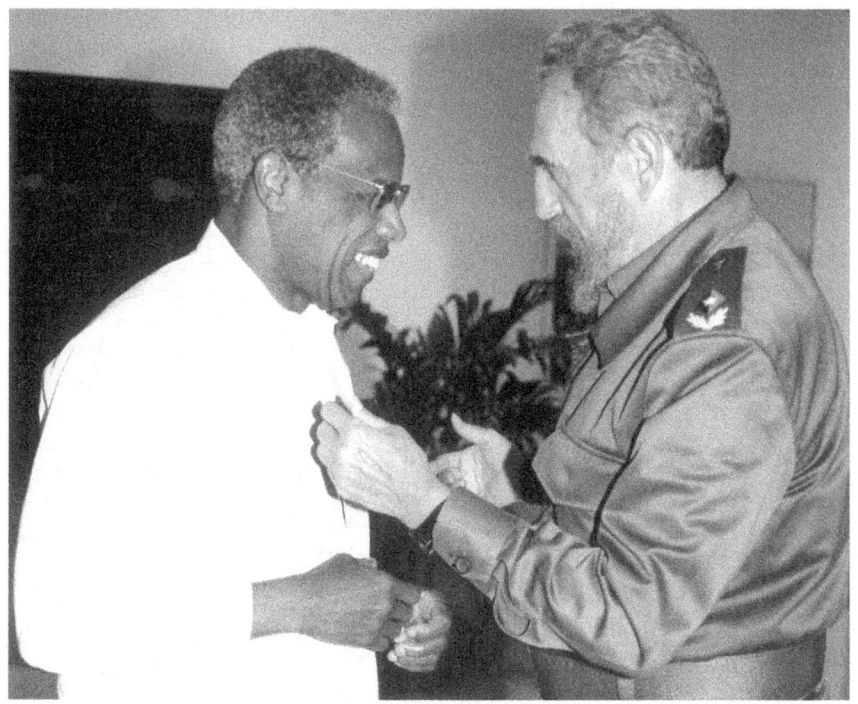

With President Fidel Castro of Cuba, May 2002

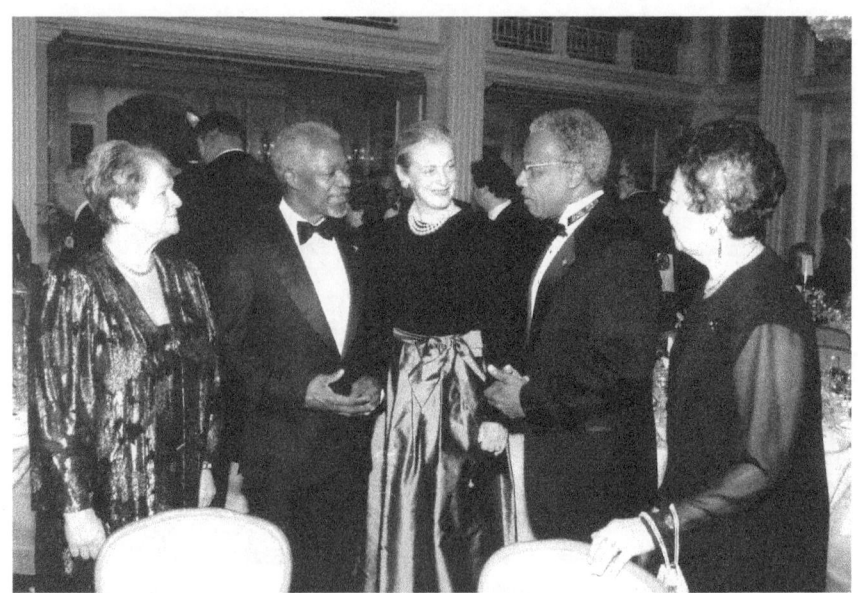

With (from left to right) Dr Brundtland, Kofi Annan, Mrs Annan, Lady Alleyne, 2002

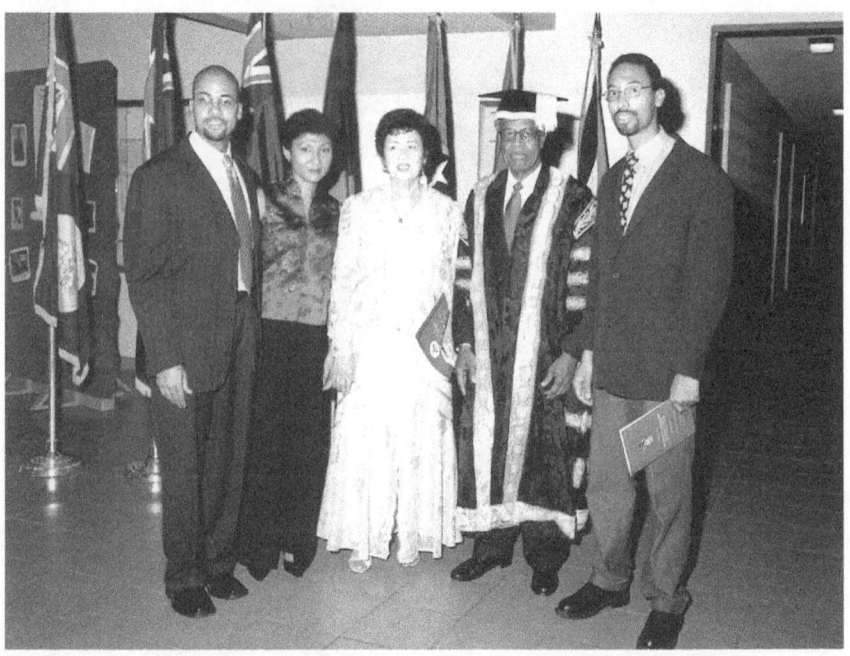

With my family (from left to right), Adrian, Carol, Sylvan and Andrew, at my installation as chancellor of the University of the West Indies, November 2003

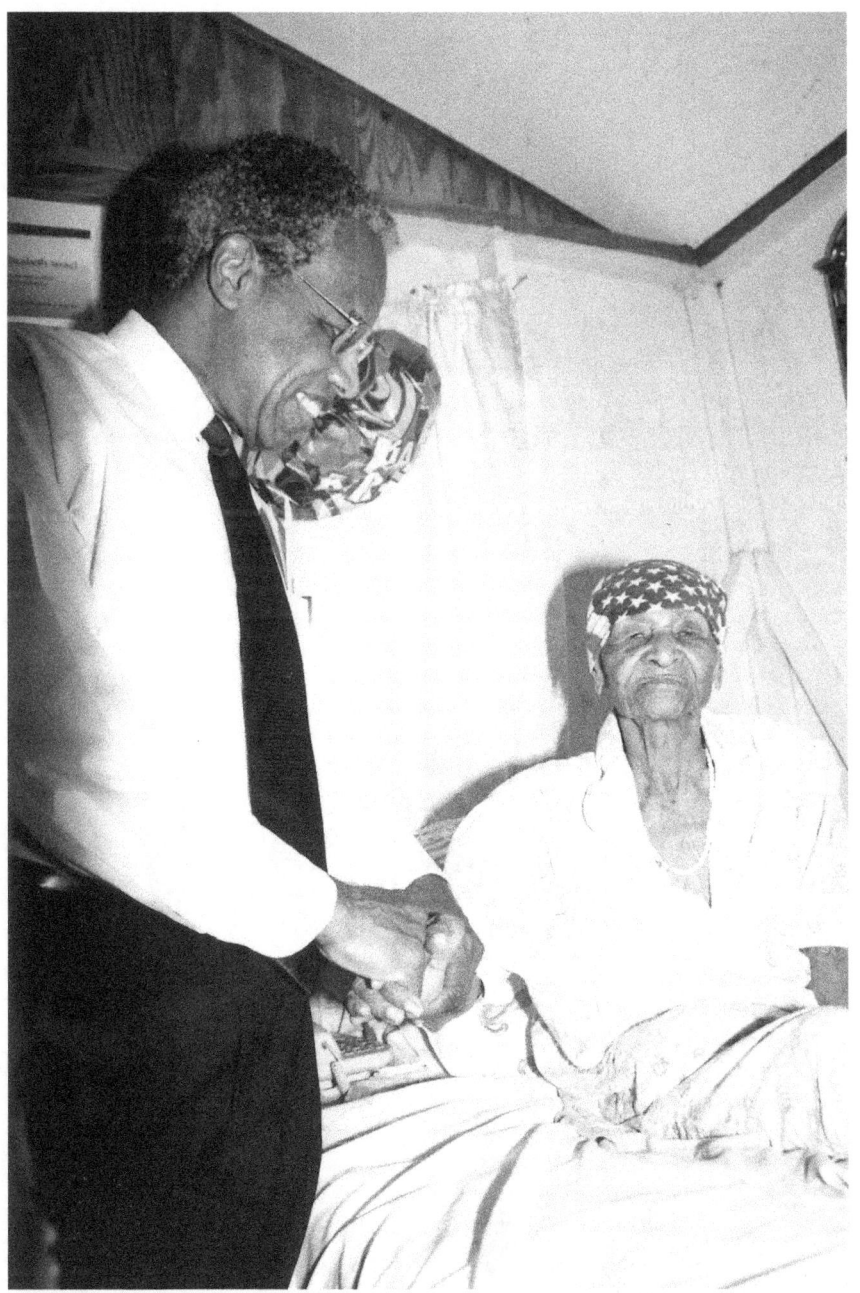
Greeting world's oldest woman, Elizabeth "Ma Pampo" Israel, 127 years old, Dominica, 2002

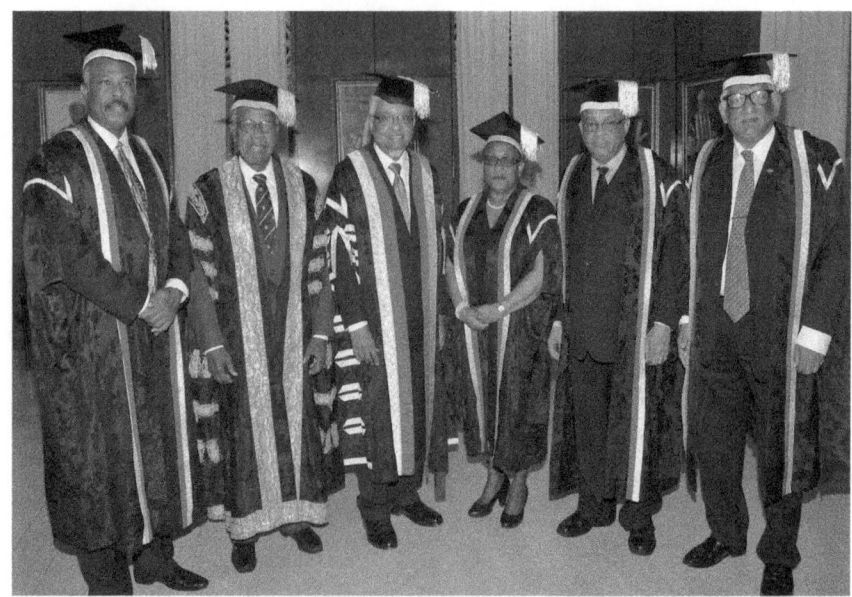

With (from left to right) Sir Hilary Beckles, pro-vice-chancellor and principal, Cave Hill campus; Professor Nigel Harris, vice chancellor; Professor Hazel Simmons McDonald, pro-vice-chancellor and principal, Open Campus; Professor Archibald Mc Donald, pro-vice-chancellor and principal, Mona campus; Professor Clement Sankat, pro-vice-chancellor and principal, St Augustine campus at Mona, Jamaica, 2013

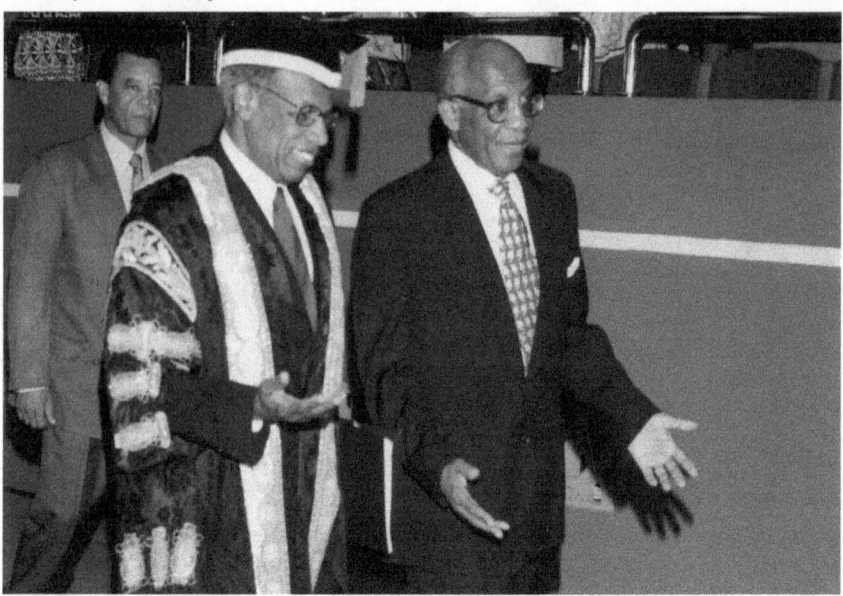

With Sir Clifford Husbands, governor general of Barbados, 2009

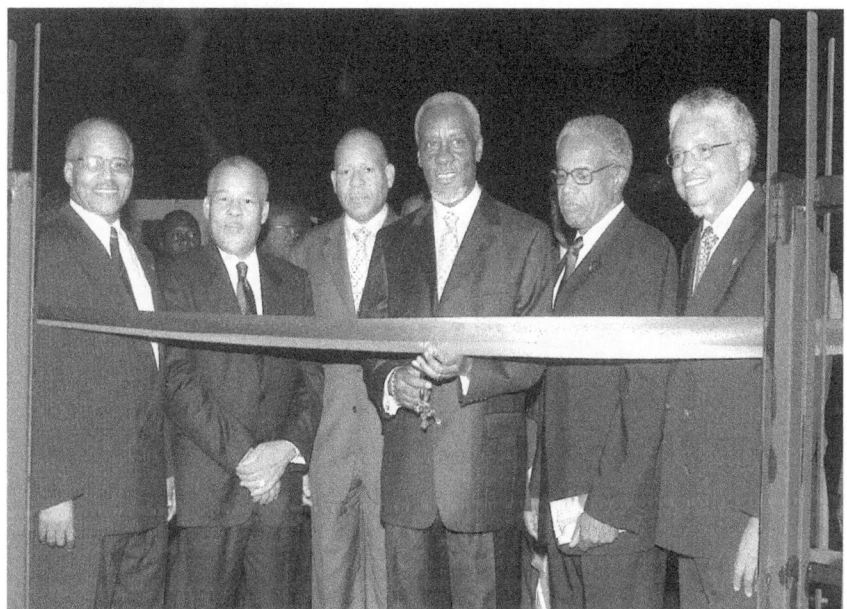

With (from left to right) Professor Kenneth Hall, Prime Minister Owen Arthur (Barbados), Prime Minister Patrick Manning (Trinidad and Tobago), the Honourable P.J. Patterson (former prime minister of Jamaica) and Vice Chancellor Nigel Harris, opening the Prime Ministers' Park, Mona, Jamaica, 2005

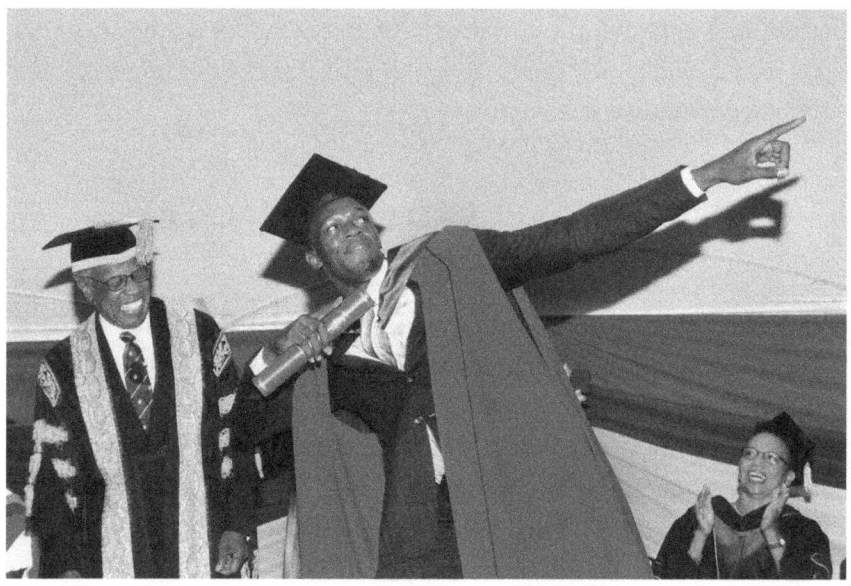

With Usain Bolt, after he received his honorary degree, Mona, Jamaica, 2014

CHAPTER 11

The Myth of Retirement

As I approached retirement in 2003, I was persuaded to seek a consultant to advise me on planning for it, as it is known that executives leaving stressful positions and suddenly finding themselves without a plan often become depressed. There were anecdotes of physical deterioration in such retirees. One result of the consultation (for which I paid handsomely) was a folder titled "The Next Phase of the Life of Sir George Alleyne". This was filled with charts, addresses and ideas as to the kind of agent I should hire and the fora at which I should aim to speak and the range of speaking fees I should expect to earn. As events unfolded, this was completely useless, and although the cornucopia of speaking fees did not materialize, I soon found myself busily occupied with a number of important and fulfilling post-retirement activities.

HIV/AIDS AND THE UN SECRETARY GENERAL'S SPECIAL ENVOY

The management of the technical cooperation for HIV/AIDS in PAHO fell within the programme for communicable diseases, which was in my area of health programmes development. I watched the evolution of the epidemic in the 1980s and 1990s, when there was despair at the high mortality, the absence of specific therapy and the fear that fuelled discrimination and much bad epidemiology, leading to unfair characterization of some groups. It soon became clear that the Caribbean was not exempt, and the regional technical cooperation was led by CAREC, which struggled against the apathy of the governments. One of the great concerns was the price of antiretroviral therapy, and we had made an attempt in PAHO to establish a revolving fund similar to that which existed for vaccines and which had played a major role in the success of the immunization programmes in the Americas. It was impossible, however, to get collaboration from the pharmaceutical companies, which insisted on selling drugs at different prices to different countries based on their appreciation of the ability to pay. The best we could achieve was to publish the information on the different prices being paid for the same drug, which we hoped would give individual countries some leverage in negotiating with the pharmaceutical companies.

But in April 2000, the Caribbean Consultative Group donors' meeting in Brussels supported inclusion of HIV/AIDS in the agenda of the June 2000 meeting of the Caribbean Group for Cooperation in Economic Development, which was convened by the World Bank in Washington. This meeting saw Caribbean Heads of Government take notice of the gravity of the epidemic.

During this meeting the Barbadian ambassador hosted a dinner at his home, at which I sat beside Prime Minister Owen Arthur. He quizzed me extensively over the epidemic and what it could mean for the countries of the Caribbean. I do not take credit for this, but on return to Barbados, Prime Minister Arthur convened a conference on HIV/AIDS in September 2000, which heard details from many sources about the size and ramifications of the epidemic. Presentations were made on the possible economic impact and the extent to which development could be derailed. Parenthetically, I have always expressed doubt about the validity of the models that were used to estimate the economic impact of the disease, although there was general agreement that reduction in human capital would have a negative impact in the region. None of the dreaded apocalyptic scenarios has developed, but, of course, the answer always is that they were prevented because of the collective actions taken. But the Cassandra analyses served their purpose of galvanizing action, and a decision was taken to establish a collaborative partnership against HIV/AIDS. This was the genesis of the Pan Caribbean Partnership against HIV/AIDS (PANCAP) which represents a multi-stakeholder effort to reach the goal of strengthening the Caribbean response to the epidemic.[1] At that time, this region was second only to sub-Saharan Africa in terms of prevalence of HIV.

I was one of the original six signatories to the Caribbean Partnership Agreement which formerly established PANCAP. The others were the prime minister of Barbados, the prime minister of St Kitts and Nevis, the secretary general of CARICOM, the executive director of UNAIDS, and the founder and coordinator of the Caribbean network of people living with HIV/AIDS(CRN+). PANCAP, ably led by a coordinating unit housed in CARICOM, has been broadened to include almost every organization involved in HIV in the Caribbean and has been successful in mobilizing resources for a Caribbean-wide response to the epidemic. It has been lauded by UNAIDS as an international best practice and mentioned as such by the secretary general of the United Nations.

In December 2002, at the celebration dinner of the PAHO centennial, I sat beside Kofi Annan, then UN secretary general. At about 9:30 p.m., when there had been much toasting and recognition of the regional health heroes, Mr Annan turned to me and said, "George, I would like you to be my special envoy for HIV/AIDS in the Caribbean." All I could say was "Certainly, sir, it would be an honour." I had no clue as to what was involved, but he continued to explain that Peter Piot, the executive director of UNAIDS, would brief me. Of course, the suggestion had originated with Peter.

Thus, in January 2003, I was officially designated United Nations Secretary General's Special Envoy for HIV/AIDS in the Caribbean. Special envoys were selected on the basis of their special competence, their technical expertise, their visibility in the international arena and their knowledge of a specific region. They were to work closely with UNAIDS and had advocacy at the country level as their main function. Originally there were four of us – for the Caribbean, Europe, Africa and Asia.

At this time, HIV/AIDS continued to represent a major problem for the Caribbean and the prevalence was still second only to that found in sub-Saharan Africa. The first cases were described in Haiti, Jamaica, and Trinidad and Tobago in the early 1980s, and the adult HIV prevalence rate was at that time about 2.3 per cent. There were approximately half a million persons in the wider Caribbean infected with the virus and about 20 per cent of these were in the CARICOM countries.

There are many social and cultural factors which contributed to the spread of the disease. Throughout the Caribbean, early sexual intercourse was common in boys and girls, and teenage pregnancy was frequent. Early sexual practices and various social norms lead to behaviour which was conducive to the increased risk of HIV infection. The gender inequalities so pervasive in many aspects of Caribbean life contributed to the increasing prevalence among young women. The environment also made for large numbers of vulnerable groups, such as men who have sex with men, and commercial sex workers, many of whom travelled extensively throughout the Caribbean to ply their trade.

The theme underpinning much of my work as special envoy was related to stigma and discrimination. I made numerous presentations to various groups on the relevance of stigma and discrimination to impeding the control of the epidemic. I discussed the nature of stigma and discrimination in numerous fora as it was directed against persons living with HIV/AIDS as well as those whose lifestyle was thought to make them more likely to develop HIV/AIDS – namely men who have sex with men. While it was possible to gain some acceptance of the view that it was almost inhuman and certainly unchristian to discriminate against persons with one particular disease, it was virtually impossible to shake the majority of those who attached a moral connotation to the practice of men having sex with men. Indeed, English-speaking CARICOM countries are the only ones in the hemisphere with laws on their books outlawing anal intercourse between consenting adults. I addressed faith-based organizations, civil society groups, national policymakers, but there was an almost implacable resistance to change of the view that the society would deteriorate rapidly if it accepted individuals' freedom to have intercourse in the manner they desired. Part of the unwillingness of political leaders to tackle the antiquated laws against buggery was the fear of public opposition which might lead to loss of political power. In addition to speaking against stigma and discrimination, I tried to stimulate enthusiasm for generating data on its prevalence and its social correlates. Many – myself included – spoke passionately about the need for reducing stigma and discrimination without any benchmark of progress.

It is difficult to get data on stigma in the Caribbean, but such data as there are show that it does exist in virulent form and may prevent as many as THIRTY per cent of women who know they are HIV positive from disclosing their HIV status even to their partners, and in some cases, they become pregnant more than once. There are well-validated accounts of persons being shunned, ostracized and abused when it was known or suspected that they were suffering from AIDS. This stigma directed against the person with AIDS in large measure derives from the fact that the disease is seen as being associated with sex and immorality, and in particular from the belief that much of the spread of AIDS is or was due to homosexual practices. Our concern about stigma is based not only on human rights considerations, but also on the fact that the stigma associated with the disease serves to drive the epidemic underground, prevents persons from coming forward for treatment even when it is available and reduces our possibility of curtailing the spread of disease. Stigma leads to the individual withdrawing from economically productive activities and therefore has an impact on the national economy. Perhaps the fear of contagion is basic to the human concern for preservation. Perhaps it is the witches' brew of sex, blood and, at one stage, the inevitability of death that has made HIV/AIDS a particular focus for stigma and discrimination.

This concern for discrimination also led to involvement in the programme of champions for change in which PANCAP sought to identify prominent individuals who would be outspoken advocates for societal change. These champions included sportsmen and women, businessmen and politicians, who lent their voices to the need for societal change in the way HIV/AIDS was regarded. I always respected and congratulated the groups of people living with HIV/AIDS, as I would postulate that partnerships and mutual support allowed their voices to be heard in the places where decisions were made, especially about resource allocation.

I involved the business sector through the Caribbean Business Coalition and could persuade the organization that its involvement in HIV/AIDS activities was not only a part of corporate social responsibility but good for business as well. Formal involvement of the Caribbean business sector was important, as through it there could be direct input into decisions of the Caribbean Heads of Government.

Funding was a perennial problem, and the national resources available were insufficient, given the magnitude of the epidemic. There were several external sources of funding, but one of the most significant was the World Bank. A recent review of its Caribbean funding shows that over two decades a total of US$131.86 million was disbursed to the CARICOM countries, with the largest amount of US$50.15 million going for two successive projects to Barbados.[2] World Bank support went beyond financing, and it used its convening power to strengthen cooperation in the region. Much of the credit for World Bank involvement in the Caribbean must go to one of its staff members, Dr Patricio Marquez.

The media obviously represent a significant channel for changing behaviour and attitudes. In 2016, the Caribbean Broadcast Media Partnership on HIV/AIDS (CBMP) was formed, uniting top broadcasters from twenty-five countries to provide a coordinated media response to the epidemic. The broadcasters used a variety of platforms to disseminate information on HIV in different formats. I chaired its independent board of trustees, to which the steering committee reported. Most of the drive and success of the partnership has been due to the enthusiasm and commitment of its executive director, Dr Allyson Leacock.

My final major activity was to organize, in collaboration with Rose-Marie Bell-Antoine, professor of law at the University of the West Indies, a conference on HIV and human rights to explore the relevant legal and policy perspectives in the Caribbean.[3] The participants involved a wide range of stakeholders – politicians, academics, civil society, people living with HIV, trade unionists and the private sector. The goal was to help to remove the legal frameworks that favoured homophobia and discrimination against people living with HIV. The underlying thesis was that there were human rights challenges that prevented an appropriate response to the epidemic. In the majority of Caribbean countries, there was no legal protection against HIV-related discrimination, and same-sex activities among consenting adults was criminalized.

The political relevance was highlighted by the then acting prime minister of Barbados, Freundel Stuart, who expanded on the notion of human rights: "The sense which I think is most appropriate for our present purposes is that in which the use of the word right connotes the existence of a duty of someone else to make claims to that right effective." He emphasized the need for the abuses of human rights to be made known.

> The word discriminate means no more than "to treat unfavorably because of". Persons living with HIV can only legitimately allege discrimination if they can prove that, in their particular case, their status was contemplated either directly or indirectly and therefore fueled an unjust or unfavorable decision or situation. If the rights of the person living with HIV or AIDS are to awaken a correlative duty in others, that duty can be discharged more effectively if those called to it are not only aware of the duty but also aware of what its effective discharge will entail.

This notion of the responsibility of the individual to make known the discrimination was intensely debated. The lawyers were firm in the applicability of the notion of human rights to the HIV problem, and one said,

> Today it is an incontrovertible fact that the language of human rights constitutes the core of the universe of discourse by which we make critical assessments of the moral legitimacy of states and their treatment of citizens. This language helps us to determine the grounds for international intervention into certain situations in order to rescue some citizens or groups of certain states from torture, hunger, starvation and so on. Put differently, human rights norms establish the moral ground for action where such action is imperative to save the lives of other human beings.

Some agreed that the denial of rights that existed represented failure of the region's parliaments to act, in which case it would rest with the courts to adjudicate on the constitutionality of the current laws and protect the fundamental rights of citizens. The presentations of people living with HIV served to emphasize the degree of discrimination that existed. The intense debate emphasized for me the fact that constitutions and laws are expressions of the ideas and prejudices of human beings at a particular time. Arguments on the applicability of one or other aspect of the constitution on the basis of original intent or to assume immutability was not conducive to the good governance of states that were constantly in a process of being perfected.

In 2010, I ceased being the United Nation secretary's special envoy, and Dr Eddie Greene was appointed to fill that role. I was pleased not only because of Dr Greene's competence but also because the secretary general felt that the situation in the Caribbean was such as to merit the continuation of the role of special envoy. Dr Greene had retired as assistant secretary general of CARICOM with responsibility for health and social development. He had been instrumental in the formation and subsequent development of PANCAP and had played a significant role in the negotiations for lowering the prices of antiretroviral drugs for the Caribbean.

HEALTH AND HUMAN DEVELOPMENT

My interest in health and human development had its genesis while I was professor of medicine. I was convinced that health of people was important for the welfare of a society in its many dimensions. Initially I was concerned with the impact of health on economic growth, and I wrote a review paper entitled "Health and Development", which I submitted to the local *Journal of Social and Economic Research*. It was rejected, and the reviewer made the comment that the paper "contained an interesting germ of an idea". The paper was subsequently published when I came to PAHO. I still entertained the idea of health being linked somehow to development, which I equated then with economic growth, so I telephoned Sir Arthur Lewis, the first vice chancellor of the University of the West Indies and a Nobel laureate in economics, who was then at Princeton, and asked if he could think of ways to link social indicators such as health to some measure of development. He listened politely and then said simply, "I know nothing about this. I suggest you consult someone like Burton Weisbrod." Weisbrod was an economist who had worked in St Lucia on the impact of schistosomiasis and parasitic diseases on economic development. Interestingly, Weisbrod and his colleagues concluded with many caveats that economic development was not being importantly retarded by parasitic disease. They were appropriately cautious in view of the established finding that high prevalence of disease was positively correlated with low income wherever the relationship was studied.

In 1989, I was invited to give the Eric Williams Memorial Lecture, which was an honour, as this had been given previously by such persons as Javier Pérez de Cuellar, the secretary general of the United Nations, Sir Arthur Lewis, and Enrique Iglesias, the president of the Inter-American Development Bank. I chose the topic of "Health and Development" and sought to establish the link between the state of health in the Caribbean and economic performance, and vice versa between the level of economic growth and health. In defining development, I referred to the statement by Dr Williams, "Development has a face – and that is the face of man", and the published lecture series is now entitled *The Face of Man*. The lecture was well received, and parenthetically, I have the signal honour of being the only person to be asked to give this prestigious lecture twice. As director of PAHO, I was able to simulate work in this area.

Then I became fascinated with the work of Mahbub ul Haq, the distinguished Pakistani economist who pointed out that economic growth was not sufficient for improvement of the country's well-being in several dimensions and elaborated the notion of human development.[4] Human development essentially embraces economic growth, education and health. I have said frequently that this formulation is reminiscent of the nursery rhyme "Early to bed, early to rise, makes a man healthy, wealthy and wise" – the last three being the main constituents of human development.

I have spoken and written on the relation of health to human development on several occasions and in several fora. Subsequent to that first Eric Williams lecture, I would expand on the relationship, indicating the nexus between health and other aspects of human development. For example, health and education are critical inputs into the formation of the human capital that is crucial for economic growth. The comparison between health and education as inputs for investment for economic growth fascinated me, and I would bewail the fact that whereas there were appropriate indicators for education, there were none for health. I would plead for the development of some "vulgar metric" for health similar to the use of years of schooling as a proxy for education.[5]

Most recently I have combined my concern for non-communicable diseases (NCDs) with human development, and prior to the elaboration of the sustainable development goals, when the world was discussing the possible scenarios post 2015, along with several colleagues I co-authored a paper "Embedding NCDs in the Post-2015 Human Development Agenda".[6] I saw human development being sustained by a triple helix of social, economic and environmental domains or strands. The concept of such a helix had been proposed by Achim Steiner of the UN Environment Programme, and I found it more appropriate as a representation of what sustained human development than the pillars which had hitherto been the dominant concept and portrayal. I would propose that health was an integral part of the social strand of the helix, and NCDs were a critical determinant of health. In addition, health was also an indicator of human development. I proposed that health was one of the capabilities essential for maintaining the integrity of the social domain. I continue to emphasize that the frequent use of development without qualification is an indication of the dominance of economic thinking, and that one should not leave the lists to the economists in this field.

I was proud when the Health Economics Unit in the St Augustine campus was renamed the Sir George Alleyne Health Economics Unit in recognition of the attention I have paid to the link between health and the economy over the years.

THE CHALLENGE OF NON-COMMUNICABLE DISEASES

The prevention and control of NCDs, principally cardiovascular disease, diabetes, cancer and chronic respiratory disease, have represented a major challenge for me for most of my professional life. First was the challenge of having to deal with them as a personal care physician, and as a nephrologist, I saw the devastating result of hypertension and diabetes on the kidney. The problems of chronic disease fell within my area in PAHO, but more recently my concern has been for garnering global attention for these diseases, which are the world's major killers.

Health was among the various topics discussed when the CARICOM Heads of Government met in Nassau in 2001. During one of the meetings, Eddie Greene, at that time assistant secretary general in CARICOM, phoned me during the meeting of our executive committee to ask my opinion as to how the final declaration should be entitled, and I recommended "The Health of the Region is the Wealth of the Region", obviously influenced by Adam Smith's *The Wealth of Nations*. The heads accepted the title and called for the establishment of a task force "to propel health to the centre of the development agenda". They recognized the importance of NCDs and HIV/AIDS and referred to the Caribbean Cooperation in Health as a continuing framework for health action.

I had been co-chair of one of the working groups – Health, Economic Growth and Poverty Reduction – of the Commission on Macroeconomics and Health established by the director general of WHO and chaired by the distinguished economist Jeffrey Sachs.[7] One of Jeffrey's ideas as a follow-up to the commission's work was to establish regional commissions. I persuaded Sergio Spinacci, who was the staff person in WHO responsible for macroeconomics and health, that funding for the cognate activity in the Caribbean as proposed by Sachs should go towards this task force, as was mandated by the CARICOM Heads of Government. The success of the task force, now renamed the Commission on Health and Development,[8] was in large measure due to the enthusiasm of Eddie Greene in CARICOM and the indefatigable support of Veta Brown, who was then the PAHO Caribbean programme coordinator in Barbados. The commissioners were decided upon by myself as chair and Eddie Greene and were a mixture of distinguished public health professionals and economists. The work was done through a series of working papers and face-to-face meetings to some of which I invited experts such as Dean Jamison and Alister McIntyre. Dean Jamison, as a former economist at the World Bank, was responsible for writing the famous 1993 World Development Report on Investing in Health. Alister McIntyre is one of the most distinguished Caribbean economists and a former vice chancellor of the University of the West Indies. The report of the commission was well received in the Caribbean, and its key message was that there were three major health problems the Caribbean faced – the NCDs and obesity, HIV/AIDS, and the health consequences of violence.

Alister had advised that the report would have the desired impact only if it was presented to the various cabinets of the Caribbean countries in addition to the conferences of the CARICOM Heads of Government. This I did in Belize, Jamaica, St Vincent, St Kitts and Nevis, Antigua and Barbuda, Dominica, Surinam, Grenada, and directly to the prime ministers of the Bahamas, and Trinidad and Tobago. In the Jamaica meeting, I was accompanied by Terrence Forrester, and in some of the others by Veta Brown. Two other commissioners, Compton Bourne and James Hospedales, made the presentation in Guyana. My presentation in Barbados was remarkable. Prime Minister Arthur organized a special meeting of the cabinet and pointed out that he had never before entertained a special presentation to his cabinet by other than a minister. I emphasized the critical nature of the major health problems and the seminal role of the political directorates in addressing them. I pointed out that the responsibility lay with the government as a whole and not uniquely with the minister of health. In each case I emphasized the need for leadership by the heads of government.

I presented the report to the Meeting of the Conference of the CARICOM Heads of Government in 2005. The heads were enthusiastic about the findings, and Prime Minister Arthur got to his feet after the applause and pointed out that the commonality of problems meant that the Caribbean should build on its traditional collective approach to health and examine the feasibility of a Caribbean-wide health insurance scheme. With the impending increases in movement of people, chronic conditions required that there be insurance coverage in all countries. Compton Bourne as president immediately offered support from the Caribbean Development Bank for this initiative. Parenthetically, many years later in spite of various consultations, CARICOM has not yet got agreement on how or if this insurance scheme should be implemented. Several of my colleagues, especially commissioners and many in CARICOM, were pleased with the result, but I was less so, as I could not see any action that would take the agenda forward.

The follow-up to the report was placed before the next Heads of Government meeting held in St Kitts and Nevis in 2006, and I was convinced that my presentation should include a specific "ask".

That meeting was a special one for another reason. As chancellor of the university, I had been having some difficult discussions with Prime Minister Manning of Trinidad and Tobago about one of our senior staff, whom he wished the university to dismiss. The university's position was that it could not dismiss a staff member because one of our member governments was concerned about his politics. Finally, it was agreed that the vice chancellor, Nigel Harris, and I would meet with him and three of the other heads of government to try to fashion a solution. Before that meeting, however, Mr Manning and I met at the margins of the governor general's cocktail reception after the formal opening of the meeting of heads – actually in the GG's garden – and he repeated his position as regards the university matter. I thanked him and repeated my position. This was an occasion for a morbid comment by Edwin Carrington, CARICOM secretary general, who was the only other person privy to our conversation. In thanking Mr Manning, I said that the university would have to stand by its position, and as to the final result, I was untroubled, as in the words of the well-known hymn, "It Was Well with My Soul". Mr Manning said something similar. At which Edwin pointed out that that hymn was a favourite for funerals, and it did not augur well for a solution to the matter under discussion.

But continuing the conversation, I referred to the findings of the commission which I would be presenting the following day. I noted the gravity of the problem mainly of cardiovascular disease and diabetes in Trinidad and Tobago and asked him to convene a national consultation on the chronic diseases and also to invite his colleague Heads to a Summit in Port of Spain to craft a regional response. These were matters on which we were both happy to agree.

After my presentation to the heads on the following day in plenary, I stressed this time not only the magnitude of the problem but the need for collective action. True to his word, Mr Manning raised his hand, complimented me warmly on the presentation and indicated that he would convene a national consultation on chronic non-communicable diseases in Trinidad and Tobago later that year, and then he invited his colleague heads to a summit in Port of Spain as soon after as possible. Parenthetically, when we met that evening to discuss the university matter, there was hard and vigorous bargaining, but eventually we found a mutually satisfactory solution. I was left with considerable regard for Mr Manning and convinced that he was a genuine regionalist. The next morning, we had a most amicable discussion on the boat over to Nevis for the Caucus of Heads.

The national consultation was convened in Port of Spain at the Crown Plaza Hotel later that year and was attended by a large number of local and foreign participants, including Dr Jerome Walcott, the minister of health of Barbados. It was addressed by Mr Manning himself, and there were impressive presentations on obesity by Shiriki Kumanike from Pennsylvania and on tobacco by Prabhat Jha from Toronto as well as by local Caribbean participants. That evening I spoke with Mr Manning by telephone (he was leaving the gym), and he asked me what he could do as a follow-up. My advice was that the single most effective action he could take was to raise taxes on tobacco. He asked for the justification, and Prabhat Jha rapidly prepared a single sheet showing the health and economic benefits of raising tobacco taxes. This was given to Mr Manning, and in his next budget speech a couple weeks later, he proceeded to raise tobacco taxes.

Given the success of the national consultation, it was imperative that a summit be convened. It was Eddie Greene again at CARICOM who pushed the agenda, as it had to be convened under CARICOM auspices. There was a basic background document to be written, for which I prepared the first draft with input from James Hospedales and Rudy Cummings. Funding had to be sought to bring the various international participants to Trinidad and Tobago. Dr Roses, then director of PAHO, was helpful, the WHO and the World Bank agreed to participate, and the Government of Trinidad and Tobago provided the venue and facilitated the meeting, but there was still need for substantial additional funding. I knew that the prime minister of Canada was due to visit the Caribbean in the near future, so I suggested that Prime Minister Douglas of St Kitts and Nevis write to him and ask for support. I drafted the letter, which I shared with Eddie Greene, and Prime Minister Douglas sent it to Prime Minister Harper. My Canadian colleagues told me that they were amazed by the rapidity with which the instructions came from the Prime Minister's Office that the request be supported. I do not recall the exact amount provided, but I think it was of the order of Can$300,000.

The summit was convened at the Crown Plaza Hotel in Port of Spain on 15 September 2007 with Prime Minister Owen Arthur as chair, since he was chair of CARICOM, and it was addressed by Prime Minister Manning, Prime Minister Douglas, who gave the lead presentation, and representatives of WHO, PAHO, and the World Bank, as well as myself and experts in NCDs such as Professors Prabhat Jha and Philip James. One of the indications of the timeliness of the summit and its importance was the fact that Prime Minister Golding of Jamaica made it his first trip out of the country after his election. Heads or senior officials from all the CARICOM countries attended. One of the notable interventions was by Prime Minister Gonsalves from St Vincent and the Grenadines, who called for a "wellness revolution" in the Caribbean. The historic declaration from the summit, "Uniting to Prevent and Control Chronic Noncommunicable Diseases", was duly constructed with input from many sources – James Hospedales, Eddie Greene, CARICOM staff, myself and others.

Mr Manning deserves much of the credit for the elevation of NCDs to the global level. After the summit, I mentioned to him and in several places that NCDs deserved the same level of attention that had been accorded to HIV and merited consideration at the level of the Security Council or the UN General Assembly. Second to Mr Manning, I would place Eddie Greene, the CARICOM assistant secretary general, in whose portfolio this matter fell, and he should be thanked for his active and enthusiastic support. Mr Manning referred to Eddie Greene and myself as the "spin twins", perhaps in reference to the famous duo of Sonny Ramadin and Alfred Valentine, two famous spin bowlers who were among the architects of West Indian prowess in test cricket in the 1950s and immortalized in Kitchener's calypso after a famous victory at Lord's as "those little pals of mine". There were subsequently three regional events of relevance to moving the NCD agenda forward in 2009: the Hemispheric Summit of the Americas, the Thirtieth Meeting of the Conference of CARICOM Heads of Government, and the Commonwealth Heads of Government Meeting.

The Hemispheric Summit of the Americas, Trinidad and Tobago, 9 April 2009

One of the paragraphs from the final communiqué reads as follows:

> We are convinced that we can reduce the burden of noncommunicable diseases through the promotion of comprehensive and integrated preventive and control strategies at the individual family community national and regional levels and through collaborative programmes, partnerships and policies supported by governments, the private sector, the media civil society organizations, communities and relevant regional and international partners. We therefore reiterate our support for the PAHO Regional Strat-

egy and Plan of Action on an integrated approach to the prevention and control of chronic diseases including diet, physical activity, and health. We also commit to measures to reduce tobacco consumption, including, where applicable, in the WHO Framework Convention on Tobacco Control.

Liliendaal Resolution of the Thirtieth Meeting of the Conference of CARICOM Heads of Government, Guyana, July 2009

Prime Minister Douglas, lead prime minister for health in the CARICOM quasi-cabinet, was unable to attend that meeting of heads in Guyana, and I was asked to present the main health issues. The topic came up on the agenda late in the day, so I dealt with one issue. I asked the heads to promote a United Nations Special assembly on NCDs and also asked that the forthcoming meeting of the Commonwealth Heads of Government support such a call.

The resolution reads as follows:

> The Conference under the heading "Realizing the Nassau Declaration of 2001: The Health of the Region is the Wealth of the Region.
>
> *Supported* the plans for the follow-up to the Port of Spain Declaration 2007, "Uniting to stop the epidemic of chronic noncommunicable diseases, including elevating the Caribbean experience to the global level;
>
> Agreed to advocate for a special UNGASS on NCDs and include NCDs within the M&E system for the MDGs (NB MDG #6) and to request that this issue be placed on the agenda of the meeting of the Commonwealth Heads of Government (CHOGM) to be held in Trinidad and Tobago in November 2009.

Commonwealth Heads of Government, November 2009

Mr Manning as host prime minister had much influence on the outcome, and there was a special declaration on NCDs, one paragraph of which reads as follows: "We further call for a summit on NCDs to be held in September 2011 under the auspices of the United Nations General Assembly in order to develop strategic responses to these diseases and their repercussions."

It was fortuitous that the meeting of the Hemispheric Summit of Heads of Government and the meeting of the Commonwealth Heads of Government were being held in Trinidad and Tobago in 2009. Mr Manning gave me his assurance that NCDs would figure in both. His sherpa for both was Luis Alberto Rodriguez, an experienced diplomat whom I was careful to brief on NCDs, and I know that he received specific relevant instructions from Mr Manning himself.

It is of interest that Prime Minister Douglas had presented the work of the Caribbean at the Commonwealth Heads of Government meeting in Kampala in 2007, but the NCDs never got the attention it did in Port of Spain, and this was obviously due to Mr Manning's influence.

Then in September 2009, in his presentation to the UN General Assembly, Mr Manning said the following:

> We are firmly of the view that noncommunicable diseases demand heightened attention by the international community at this time. It is forecasted that by 2020, NCDs will account for about 73 per cent of global deaths and 60 per cent of the global burden of diseases. We join the call for indicators on noncommunicable diseases and injuries to be integrated into the core millennium development goals MDGs monitoring and evaluation system.
>
> We have taken on board this matter at the level of CARICOM and, indeed, we held a special regional summit in Port of Spain on chronic noncommunicable diseases in 2007. I now propose to this August assembly that a special session of the United Nations General Assembly on noncommunicable diseases be convened at the earliest opportunity.

The stars were then in alignment, and there were several contributors to the realization of the historic 2011 UN meeting. WHO was a major advocate, especially Dr Ala Alwan, assistant director general, who was instrumental in having it placed before many regional meetings, including that in the eastern Mediterranean. There was a UN Economic and Social Council resolution, and my recollection is of briefing one of the delegates, the ambassador of Barbados, Christopher Hackett, who was an ardent advocate for the special assembly.

The matter was discussed and supported by the meetings of CARICOM Foreign Ministers and the Caribbean ambassadors in New York were collectively energized to lobby for the meeting. It is proper here to recognize the valuable role played by Karen Sealey, who provided information and guidance in briefing meetings with the CARICOM ambassadors in New York. It was a pleasure to note the high regard with which she was held and how her counsel was valued.

Both the Port of Spain Declaration and the UN high-level meeting refer to the involvement of civil society. I had accepted to be patron of the Healthy Caribbean Coalition, an umbrella Caribbean civil society organization focused on NCDs, which was founded by Professor Sir Trevor Hassell, a distinguished Barbadian cardiologist. In May 2009, during the World Health Assembly, Ann Keeling, executive director of the International Diabetes Federation, arranged for me to have lunch with Martin Sillink, an Australian paediatrician and president of the federation. We discussed the way forward, and I expressed the wish to see NCDs reach the level of the Security Council, but he was more realistic and pointed out that a meeting of the UN General Assembly was far more practical. Subsequently that week I was a member of a panel organized by the International Diabetes Federation to discuss the critical nature of having political support for NCDs and to announce the formation of the NCD Alliance, an alliance of the International Diabetes Federation, the World Heart Federation, the International Union against Cancer, and the Tuberculosis and Lung Association. In his opening remarks, Martin pointed out the gravity of the epidemic and said that he had a dream that NCDs would one day be considered at a high political level such as the United Nations. When my turn came to speak, I opened my remarks thus: "I am blessed to live to hear a white man named Martin say I have a dream." The audience erupted, and it was some time before the laughter and applause subsided.

The high-level meeting was convened at the United Nations in 2011 with the participation of eighty-five heads of state and issued the Political Declaration which has subsequently been the critical backdrop to international action on NCDs. I participated in this meeting and since then have been active at the Caribbean and international level through numerous oral and written presentations in promoting the actions that must take place to make the declaration meaningful.

I have discussed NCDs at length, as this area represents one of the finest examples of collective CARICOM action to advance to the highest political level. It is now recognized in international circles that the Caribbean was a major player in focusing international attention on NCDs, and I am proud to have played a part in this effort. My role in this field was recognized when my name was attached to the chronic disease research centre in Barbados.

THE CARIBBEAN AND HEALTH SECURITY

I was a member of a Lancet Commission on investing in health whose report pointed out that the world will have to face three major threats in the immediate future: NCDs, anti-microbial resistance and the threat of pandemic influenza. I am pleased with the concern for NCDs that has continued in the Caribbean, but the other two threats need more scrutiny. The ravages of recent pandemics and that possibility of a new pandemic of influenza which will kill millions of people have led to an increased interest in global health security and the design of instruments that minimize the vulnerability of populations to health risks. I am concerned that the Caribbean countries tend to think of security in terms of the protection of borders from perpetrators of crime and violence and at a second level in terms of vulnerability to natural hazards. Until recently I did not detect enough interest in health security and less interest in global health security; although the evidence is clear that breakdown in global health security can have cataclysmic effects. The SARS epidemic of 2003 caused economic havoc principally in the more developed countries, but there is less appreciation of the magnitude of the problem that might occur if there were to be some major infectious disease outbreak in countries which depend economically on international travel. The recent epidemics of chikungunya and zika are but a glimpse of what could happen in a global pandemic.

Health security has gone through many phases.[9] First there was unilateral imposition of quarantine mainly in European ports; next there was the birth of international cooperation and the view that collective action might keep diseases like cholera away from one's country. Then, in the first half of the last century, we saw the growth of international cooperation and acceptance of the view that control of disease everywhere would be beneficial to everyone – a concept that led to the formation of the Pan American Health Organization in 1902. In the second half of the last century, there was more formalization of international cooperation which saw the birth of the World Health Organization in 1948 and the subsequent development of International Health Regulations that guide state action. The International Health Regulations, while they break the "Westphalian bargain of exclusive state authority in international affairs",[10] are hampered by the fact that there is no global or international enforcement mechanism analogous to that which exists in the states themselves. To add to this, there is increasing challenge to the international system and increased practice of multilateralism among the developed countries with new loci of intergovernmental debate and discussion such as the G8, the Global Health Security initiative with the WHO being just one of the many actors in the global health security field is another example.

The future is unclear. One possibility sees WHO assuming the power and authority to be a hegemonic figure coordinating the various actors. The precarious nature of its funding make this unlikely, and my view is that the world will see the evolution of a World Health System with leadership coming from the part of the system with the demonstrated capacity to make a difference. One may see civil society and the private sector playing critical roles in this evolution.

Small states such as those in the Caribbean are in a particularly difficult position. WHO and the United Nations represent fora in which they have a voice and can influence events. Reduction of the influence of the United Nations and WHO will impact negatively on the health security capacity of small states whose only recourse may be the formation and strengthening of their own blocs to argue their case effectively and evolve forms of mutual cooperation. The mutuality of interests in these matters exists in the Caribbean, and it has institutions which can help to strengthen global health security such as the Caribbean Public Health Agency, the Caribbean Disaster Emergency Response Agency and the University of the West Indies. It is critical that the degree of attention given to health security is as keen as that given to such areas as natural hazards and crime and violence, important though these may be. I was therefore pleased to note recently that the Caribbean Public Health Agency has been in the lead in establishing the basis for a CARICOM health security agenda and has been actively promoting the inclusion of the CARICOM countries in the Global Health

Security Agenda. This is a partnership of nations, international organizations and various stakeholders to address the threat of global spread of infectious disease.

JOHNS HOPKINS BLOOMBERG SCHOOL OF PUBLIC HEALTH

In spring 2003, I received a call from Al Sommer, dean of the school, inviting me to join the faculty. I had previously been a member of the school's advisory board and had given the occasional lecture as well as a convocation address. I met him at the school in Baltimore and pointed out that I could not entertain a full-time appointment. To which Al replied puckishly, "George, the difference between my full-time and my part-time faculty is that the part-timers travel part of the time." With that, I agreed to join the faculty as a visiting professor in the Department of International Health.

This department was started by Carl Taylor, and when I met him, I reminded him of our meeting on the plane from Chiang Mai to Bangkok in 1974, when he had advised me "to do something useful with my life and enter public health". His rejoinder was something along the lines that it was never too late to do something useful.

The Johns Hopkins Bloomberg School of Public Health is the oldest and largest school of public health in the world. Originally named the Johns Hopkins School of Hygiene and Public Health, it was founded by William Welch with a grant from the Rockefeller Foundation. It is said that hygiene was included in the name to emphasize research about disease, following a German tradition, and public health owed its inclusion to the English tradition of seeking practical solutions to the health of populations. The school was renamed the Johns Hopkins Bloomberg School of Public Health in 2011 in honour of Michael Bloomberg, a Johns Hopkins alumnus and mayor of New York, in recognition of his generous financial support to the school and to the university. There are ten academic departments, more than five hundred full-time and more than six hundred part-time faculty, with over two thousand students from eighty-eight countries. Its motto is "Saving lives millions at a time".

Over the past thirteen years, I have been able to renew my pleasure for teaching and mentoring young people. One of my favourite lectures was on global health, in which I would trace the development of the concern for global health and point out that this became fashionable, replacing the concept of international health. But much of what was called global health was simply international health by another name and was indeed little more than missionary health, in which health workers from the developed world went to carry out "projects" in the developing world. While this was laudable, the practice did not embrace much of the essence of global health, which I took to mean the health of the world's people with particular emphasis on reducing the health inequities which existed. I would emphasize the relevance of NCDs as a global health problem. I also enjoyed teaching a fascinating course entitled "Management Decision-making", which involves a description and discussion of the approaches senior managers should take to make rational decisions. One of the fundamentals of the course is understanding the elements of principled negotiation, and a required reading is the excellent small book by Fisher and Ury, *Getting to Yes*.[11] One of my favourite evaluations about the course was from a student who wrote that my teaching on negotiation was helpful to him when he was going through his divorce. On retiring from the school in 2017, I gave a special dean's lecture and was awarded the dean's medal. Its inscription reads, "Sir George Alleyne M.D., an inspirational leader of health diplomacy and champion of health equity."

CHAPTER 12

The Return of the Pelican
Back at the University of the West Indies

I had maintained contact with the University of the West Indies and played some part in activities such as the formation of the UWI Medical Alumni Association, and indeed was given a special award for this in 1988. Hurricane Gilbert had ravaged the Mona campus in November 1988, and seven months later, the university called a Special Convocation, attended by many of the CARICOM Heads of Government, at which it recognized distinguished graduates. I was among a group of four alumni – the others were Ewart Thomas, Edwin Carrington and Gloria Samms-Knight – who received honorary doctorates. Ewart was professor of mathematical psychology at Stanford University, Edwin was secretary general of CARICOM, and Gloria was one of the most respected Jamaican public servants of her generation. The public orator ended my citation thus: "Chancellor, for showing us all what this University can achieve and for giving us an example from its forty years of existence in terms of human excellence, we can do no more than what the Scriptures command us and 'honour a physician with the honour due unto him'."

The guest speaker was Sir Shridath Ramphal, who was not yet chancellor. He delivered a stirring address in which he made a nostalgic journey back in time, enumerated some of the challenges ahead and ended with a magnificent peroration: "Let me end then with words which have echoed through the whole history of universities and which may be heard whenever a university marks both so serious and so joyous a commemoration as that which we celebrate today; To the University of the West Indies I say for all of us – *Vivat, Floreat, Crescat*: Live, Flourish, Grow!"

In 1993, Sylvan and I attended the first Gathering of the Graduates to mark the forty-fifth anniversary of the university. It was brilliantly organized by Eddie Greene, then pro-vice-chancellor, and Cecile Clayton, and saw graduates from all parts of the world, including many heads of government, converge on Mona for a week of celebration, reminiscing and partying. There were numerous exhibitions, conferences and seminars, which all contributed to the main theme of "Unlocking the Potential". Some of the more fascinating experiences were the informal seminars and conversations animated by a mixture of recollections and opinions, especially from elder statesmen such as John Figueroa and Roy Augier, who wore their grey beards as badges of experience and authority.

In 1996, the chancellor asked me to be one of his nominees on council, and I attended my first meeting in this capacity in St Kitts and Nevis. The university celebrated its fiftieth birthday in July 1998 with a Convocation Week and a Special Awards Ceremony, at which it honoured some of its most outstanding alumni and others who had contributed to its growth and development. I gave the opening keynote address, titled "Pride in the Product". I said I was "honoured to be the mouthpiece of the many thousands of the sons and daughters of the *Pelican*, most of whom are here in spirit as we celebrate this auspicious occasion. Perhaps if we listen carefully we can hear them singing that ancient song of celebration – '*gaudeamus igitur, juvenes dum sumus*' – let us therefore rejoice while we are young – fifty years young." I was unabashedly expansive about what the university had accomplished and how it had hewed to the essence of its charter in "providing a place of education, learning and research". One of my paragraphs is just as relevant today as it was then.

> I have encouraged you like me to be triumphalistic and glory in fifty years of achievement and the recognition of the products of our University. But you will no doubt on these occasions also hear the revisionists who will tell you of the things that ought to be done and have not been done – that perhaps by now the University should have produced more than one Nobel Prize winner – that none of its scientists has found magic bullets to cure our diseases – that its students occasionally fight and cause disturbances – that

the University is not finding a place for the many thousands of West Indians qualified to enter – and that the old days were truly good! You must not challenge the truth or relevance of what they say. But you will say to them, as Martin Luther said about five hundred years ago,

> We are not what we shall be, but we are growing towards it. The process is not yet finished but it is going on. This is not the end, but it is the road. All does not yet gleam in glory, but all is being purified.

I also paid special tribute to Alister McIntyre, saying, "He is my friend, but that is not an encomium, it is a prelude to saying that there are few men for whom I have more respect and admiration – for his undoubted intellectual gifts, his commitment and for his humanness. We all owe him a lot." Alister was thinking of retiring, and I was asked if I would consider applying for his post, but I declined, as I was planning to seek re-election as director of PAHO later that year. Eventually Alister was succeeded that year by Rex Nettleford, who had been deputy vice chancellor and was the first of our graduates to be appointed vice chancellor. He brought with him vast experience of university matters, an enormous talent and a tremendous and well-deserved reputation as a scholar and an artist.

I attended several meetings of council and was struck by the manner in which Sir Shridath handled the business with dispatch. But he was an experienced chancellor, having served in that capacity in Warwick University for many years.

With the possible retirement of Rex Nettleford as vice chancellor, a joint committee of council and senate was appointed in 1999 to select a new vice chancellor, and I was asked to chair it. We winnowed down the large number of applicants to six, but after interviewing five, and reading referees' reports and candidates' vision statements, it was still impossible to reach a consensus. I had introduced a judging scheme based on having the committee members score the candidates' various competencies. In spite of much discussion and some changes in preferences, it was still impossible to reach a consensus, and the committee finally voted six to four in favour of Professor Hilary Beckles, an eminent Barbadian historian who was at that time a pro-vice-chancellor, and I reported so to an extraordinary meeting of council in July 2001.

I approached the council meeting with some trepidation, as I was well aware that despite the members agreeing to maintain confidentiality, the results of the committee's deliberations had been discussed outside the meeting. The discussion at council bordered on the acrimonious. The minister from Barbados, an ardent and vocal supporter of Beckles, was emphatic that the committee's final majority decision should be adopted, and she accused the council of rank discrimination. The majority view, however, was that such an important decision should be based on a consensus, and this prevailed, much to the minister's patent displeasure. Rex Nettleford was asked to continue as vice chancellor, and at a regular meeting of council in April 2002, a new committee was appointed to be chaired by Marshall Hall, one of the chancellor's nominees on council. Professor Hilary Beckles was appointed principal of the Cave Hill campus at this time.

Normally, knowing that Sir Shridath's second term would end in 2003, a committee would have been established by council in 2002 to conduct a search for a chancellor and make a recommendation to council for its approval in 2003. The minutes of the council of 2001 make no mention of such action, and, strangely, the council meeting of 2002 did not establish a committee to select a new chancellor. Sir Shridath announced his retirement at the annual meeting of council in April 2003, and the vice chancellor proposed that he chair a committee to select a person to be presented to council for appointment as chancellor. Lawrence Carrington approached me to ask if I would agree to my name going forward, which I did. I was not privy to the discussions of the committee, but the extraordinary meeting of council of September 2003 records that the committee unanimously agreed to propose Sir George Alleyne be appointed chancellor, and the proposal was greeted with sustained applause.

Council took the remarkable step of giving a clearer definition of the role of chancellor, since the charter was not expansive on this particular. The relevant council paper states: "We rely therefore as much on tradition and precedent as on the vision of the incumbent in shaping the expectations of the post."

Council did, however, establish some basic duties and responsibilities of the post. The chancellor was expected to provide leadership in promoting and protecting a positive image of the institution and ensure that a vision statement and a strategic plan to guide the development of the university be articulated, and monitor the implementation of said plan. One of the duties bears specific mention: "The Chancellor shall fashion and maintain a constructive and mutually supportive working relationship with the Vice Chancellor or chief executive office of the University as well as with the University registrar and other members of the senior management team while demanding accountability of them."

The chancellor was also expected to ensure that the regional focus of the university's mandate was maintained. On reflection, in light of the duties and responsibilities council assigned to the office, the appointment of the chancellor is one aspect of governance that should be revisited. As a matter of institutional governance, it may not be appropriate for the vice chancellor to chair a committee selecting a chancellor, when council expects the chancellor, if not to supervise, at least to demand accountability of the vice chancellor

THE CHANCELLORSHIP

The process of selecting the new vice chancellor was a long one, involving at least seven meetings plus numerous consultations with stakeholders, as there were excellent candidates, among whom was Hilary Beckles, a candidate the first time around and now principal of the Cave Hill campus. Another was Nigel Harris, dean of Morehouse School of Medicine in Atlanta, Georgia, a Guyanese who had studied medicine in the United States but returned to Mona for his postgraduate training. He had been one of my residents when I was professor of medicine. Eventually Marshall got the committee to arrive at a consensus that Nigel Harris should be appointed.

On reflection and in comparing Marshall's success in arriving at a consensus with my failure to do so, I reached some conclusions. First, there was less implacability now than there had been among some committee members previously. There had been changes of government, there was less political pressure at this stage, and, given the problem of the first effort, council and the committee were more disposed to allow a protracted process. I also recognize the merit of Marshall's decision not to entertain any quantitative assessment of the candidates, but to engage in an iterative process of debate and discussion until there was consensus.

The extraordinary council meeting to appoint a vice chancellor was held in Barbados in the morning of 3 December 2003, and my installation was held in the evening. I was apprehensive that the minister of education of Barbados would reopen the discussion on the process and perhaps be as vocal as his predecessor had been in the previous exercise. I approached him before the meeting, and I recall his words clearly: "Sir George, Barbados cannot rain on your parade." The meeting went smoothly, and council accepted with applause the recommendation that Nigel Harris be appointed vice chancellor. Clearly Hilary Beckles must have been disappointed, but to his great credit, he was the epitome of grace and good humour at my installation that evening, pledging in firm and unwavering terms his support and loyalty to me and the institution.

Between my selection and my installation, I reflected deeply on what it would mean that for the first time, a graduate of the university would be its head. Sir Hugh Wooding, the first West Indian chancellor, had titled his installation address "The Last of Our Beginnings", reflecting the assumption of self-reliance. My election would no doubt signal the continued affirmation that the chancellor should be from the region. But in addition, it was an indication of the maturation of the institution that its leadership should come from one of its own products. A handsome crop has its beginnings in good seed corn. There were several briefings with Rex Nettleford, the vice chancellor, who was an undergraduate with me at Mona, and the registrar, Gloria Barrett-Sobers, to acquaint me with the inner workings of the institution of which I was not aware and which I should know if I was to discharge the remit given by council.

Much of my thinking about the discharge of my duties was reflected in my installation address "Voices of the Pelican". I conceived my first responsibility as projecting the notion of the irrevocability of the Declaration of Grand Anse by the Heads of Government in 1989 that the university should remain a regional institution indefinitely. Rex was fond of saying "in perpetuity". This conviction was born of my own commitment to the regional enterprise and a strong sense that the collapse of the political adventure with unity was a failure of the preceding generation. Any failure of UWI would represent an equal or more damning blot on the escutcheon of my generation. Our university had risen from the ashes of our colonial past and was a standing monument to the conviction that such a past was now behind us.

I rhapsodized then:

> We processed this afternoon to one of my favourite pieces of music, "By the Rivers of Babylon", the musical version of Psalm 137:1–4, which is one of the most poignant expressions of lament and longing for liberation, both physical and spiritual, that I know:
>> By the rivers of Babylon, there we sat down, yea, we wept, when we remembered Zion.
>> We hanged our harps upon the willows in the midst thereof.
>> For there they that carried us away captive required of us a song; and they that wasted us required of us mirth, saying, Sing us one of the songs of Zion.
>> How shall we sing the LORD'S song in a strange land?

And I referred to "the conviction that although we too were carried away into captivity and for many a day could not really sing our song, today we can. Today we have voice, and the fact that I and many like me have a voice and can sing our song in any land is because of the University of the West Indies."

I saw the university confronting several tensions – the tension between the creation of knowledge for its own sake and the perception that was common in the Caribbean that knowledge was utilitarian – the tension between excellence for a few and general training for many. I saw the university contributing to the basic freedoms that are at the core of our Caribbean development.

> We have to produce human resources and the research to strengthen our capacity for economic growth, for improving the health of our people, for protecting our environment, for improving our stock of human and social capital and for enhancing the capacity of individuals and communities to embrace democratic principles and uphold human rights. The only concern is that these must not be seen as inimical to the constitutive value of education.

The Return of the Pelican: Back at the UWI

I called for a Caribbean tertiary education system and affirmed that our university would not be seeking hegemony but would help the Caribbean countries improve their capacity for tertiary education. I called on alumni to support the university, and I ended by affirming my love for the university and continued thus: "That love is of course sprinkled with nostalgia and laced with sentimentality. But it is also hardened by the deep and sure conviction that the actual and potential energy of my University – our university, that light from the west, represents one of the best and surest hopes for illuminating a Caribbean future that is brighter than our Caribbean present."

In my first year, I visited almost every one of our member countries, speaking to alumni and government officials, bearing the same message: that the regionality of the institution was precious cargo to be preserved for current and future generations. It is interesting to reflect now on the past fourteen years and the impact of reality on my perhaps starry-eyed vision of what a chancellor could do. I was chastened by a friend who was chancellor of an English university and who advised me that the effective role of a chancellor was to "exert influence without interfering". But for me, the remit of council seemed to imply some degree of interference.

It was also clear that it was time to revisit the governance of the institution, as the previous study had been carried out in 1994. I secured funding from the International Development Research Centre and the Commonwealth Secretariat, and council established a committee with representation from all the major stakeholders and participation by two external experts in university affairs. It was instructive and gratifying that there were no government representatives, and I took it to be a mark of confidence by governments that while such an exercise needed government input, it did not need government supervision.

The process involved interviews with all the member governments and a wide cross-section of the university community as well as the public. The first hurdle was to find an acceptable definition of *governance*, as the term was subject to numerous interpretations. Our definition was "the structures and processes through which the decisions get made that allow for the optimal functioning of the institution". When I presented our final report to council, it generated tremendous discussion over almost two days, and eventually a review committee was established under the able leadership of Joe Pereira to review our recommendations in light of the discussion.

The most important of the recommendations was in relation to the twelve countries that were designated "non-campus countries". Our committee found this term pejorative, and in addition, several heads of government told us that unless the university established physical, identifiable presences in each of the contributing territories, it would become irrelevant. It was finally agreed that these twelve countries would come under one academic umbrella and be designated as forming the Open Campus. Our committee had opted for the term "Fourth Campus", one with its own administrative structure similar to what obtained in the other three campuses, but with the caveat that many of the required back-office functions could be shared. It was interesting that as soon as the discussion turned on a physical location, there was jockeying among the countries for the site of the administrative structure. There were several decisions on the recommendations as to the size and composition of council, the value and composition of the strategy and planning committee, the formal involvement of deans and the retention of the School for Graduate Studies. Parenthetically, I argued strongly and in vain that such a school was inappropriate in our circumstances and contended that all staff should be encouraging graduate studies and graduate students.

Initially I had many concerns about the role and functioning of the council and ideas about ensuring that it not be a cipher. Given that the finance and general purposes committee could act for council and met more frequently, it was possible that council could be reduced to playing a perfunctory and almost ceremonial role. I doubt that this was what the ordinances and statues had envisaged. I was concerned that the council meetings followed a set pattern of a report by the vice chancellor which often evoked minimal comment, acceptance and noting of various reports and the statutory functions of confirming the appointments or extension of senior managers. Given the composition of council – ministers of education and senior academics – I felt that it did not provide a forum for optimal use of the talents and resources present.

I sought to include more discussion on the reports from the campus councils, commentary from the chairs of those councils and stimulated discussion on various issues on which I thought wider ventilation was useful. I expanded the meetings to two days instead of a half-day, but soon found that the level of enthusiasm for debate was only enough for one day's discussion. Given the council's mandate to the chancellor to be involved in the university's strategic plan, I was initially concerned about the nature of that exercise, as much of what was presented concentrated on the statistical analysis, with no clearly defined measurable targets and objectives or methods of verification. Coming from PAHO, where I had been involved in and committed to strategic planning and evaluation, I was discomfited at the process in our university. However, there has been significant advance over the years with the accent on defining more clearly the objectives and the locus of responsibility and reporting, and much of this has been due to the collaboration of the vice chancellors.

I am still to be convinced that our strategy and planning committee, which should be deeply involved in the strategic planning process, plays any meaningful role. In addition, I have reluctantly come to the conclusion that senior academics in general regard planning with considerable scepticism if not an exercise to be resisted.

I placed great emphasis on the reports of the audit committee and initially was amazed to find in the first ones that there was no record of any malfeasance or deviation from standard practice. Audit of the non-financial aspects of the institutions operation represented an area of vulnerability in need of constant oversight, and I am pleased to note the steady strengthening of the functions and operations of that committee, particularly under the chairmanship of Aubyn Hill, one of my nominees on council. Nevertheless, our meetings of council have improved over the years in form and content. I must pay tribute to the registrars and their staff for the considerable effort they have made in preparing for these meetings.

The statutes indicate that the chancellor shall preside over meetings of the Guild of Graduates, and it is assumed that the same function obtains now that the Guild of Graduates, since 2006, has become the UWI Alumni Association. The relevant ordinance sets out the responsibilities of the association, and on the occasions when I have presided over meetings of the association, I have stressed these, paying particular emphasis to the responsibility which speaks to alumni being benefactors of the university. I have always contended that alumni represent a critical part of the university, and over the years, I have been intimately involved in alumni affairs. I was president of the guild in 1980 and have had the privilege of receiving two Pelican Awards for my service in Jamaica and in Washington. Over the course of my chancellorship, there has been considerable advance in communicating with alumni, providing them with information, incorporating them into our formal ceremonies and developing programmes to encourage involvement even before graduation, with the idea that students are alumni in training, or, through a formal programme named STAT – "Students Today, Alumni Tomorrow".

THE VICE-CHANCELLORS

The council saw the chancellor establishing a constructive working relationship with the vice chancellor, who, according to the statutes, "shall exercise general and specific supervision over the educational arrangements of the University" and "shall maintain and promote the efficiency and good order of the University".

I have related to three vice chancellors, each very different in approach and managerial style but with whom I managed to establish a productive relationship based on open communication and mutual trust.

Rex Nettleford and I were undergraduates on campus at the same time, and he was the first of our graduates to become vice chancellor. This made for considerable ease in our relationship during the short overlap period in which he was vice chancellor. He had made the university his life and wore it on his sleeve for all the world to see. Perhaps he had two lives, as he was also the founder of the world-acclaimed National Dance Theatre Company of Jamaica. He had himself served five principals and vice chancellors, and as vice chancellor, he exercised a style of administration befitting a paterfamilias with only the absolute necessary attention to details of strategic planning and such. He had an abhorrence for asking for money, and perhaps that was the reason why the university did not have a significant endowment fund. He once stated that there was little difference between managing the university and managing the dance company, as in both one had to cope with and accommodate to a variety of prima donnas. He

The Return of the Pelican: Back at the UWI

was universally respected, loved and admired. There are numerous well-deserved laudatory descriptions of his work and tributes to him, but I extract one by Barry Chevannes, as he demitted office in 2004.

> He was there when the campus became two and then it became three. He was there during the turbulent years of student power then black power, when gown went to town and changed the nature of our interface, when we grew from an essentially residential to an essentially commuting community of scholars. He was there when the demographic profile of the campuses became national, when under the pressure of the North we semestered, when we adopted a new governance structure, he was there throughout it all, studying, encouraging, counselling, the sage optimist, incorruptibly confident in the wisdom and creative power of the Caribbean people.

And here I cite an extract from a tribute by then-prime minister of Jamaica P.J. Patterson, who was one of his contemporaries at university: "Professor Rex Nettleford is a colossal figure in the intellectual and cultural arena of the African Diaspora and deservedly so, as no other person has so single-handedly created and eloquently defined a space that our peoples are at last beginning to accept as a legitimate rendering of the collective identity."

A few years later, I presented him with the Chancellor's Medal, which is given to persons or institutions that have made outstanding contributions to the university or the Caribbean. In his acceptance speech, he revealed some of his feelings about the university.

> In its sixty years of existence there are a couple or so generations of us who can look back, praise the Lord and pass the ammunition of intellect and imagination in creative, conscious transfer of knowledge and know-how to a new generation and, through that generation, hopefully to one yet unborn. It is for this reason that I have had cause to marvel at a seemingly concerted effort in one part of this region to less-count the achievements and continuing significance of what I have always regarded as the Commonwealth Caribbean's finest gift to itself as a transforming idea of light, liberty and learning. For in providing for six or so million of our region's tenants the capacity to exercise their intellect and creative imagination, it

has helped a great many of us to know that self-empowerment comes with the capability to make definitions about self on one's own terms and to be able to proceed to action on the basis of such definitions.

I was there when Rex died suddenly in Washington, DC, in 2010, and I took his ashes back to be buried in the grounds of the University Chapel at Mona. There were numerous tributes to him, and I gave a eulogy in Washington titled "The Ammunition of Intellect and Imagination". I cite here two passages.

> He had a passion for people, a passion for perfection in whatever he did and a passion to perfect the perception of our people about their proper and rightful pride in themselves and their intrinsic worth. . . .
>
> Rex was a fervent proponent of the thesis that it is important for a people to establish an identity and some of his more eloquent passages speak to the need for the appreciation of self which must precede the self-respect that a people must have if they are to truly develop in the sense of enlarging and enhancing their capacities for living. He was racially conscious without being racist, and it was clear that for him it was necessary to appreciate the dissonance inherent in the racial and ethnic diversity that was native to the Caribbean as a pre-requisite to achieving the harmony that for Rex and many others of us is almost a holy grail. Dissonance is essential for harmony.
>
> His body was cremated, and thereby hangs a tale. I went to the crematorium to view the body and placed a coin on his chest. When asked about it subsequently, I referred to classical lore and said that the coin was to pay the boatman Cheiron to ferry him across the Styx. Failure to pay would mean that he would wander on the banks of the river for two hundred years. I repeated the account at a family gathering, whereupon my eight-year-old grandson corrected me: "Grandpa, the boatman's name is Charon. Cheiron is the centaur who was son of Titan." I was both chagrined and proud!

Nigel Harris is Guyanese, had studied medicine in the United States and came to Jamaica for his postgraduate training. After completing his postgraduate training, he went to Britain and then to the United States, eventually becoming dean of Morehouse School of Medicine in Atlanta, Georgia. He had had a brilliant academic career and was widely and highly respected

The Return of the Pelican: Back at the UWI

in his professional field, especially for his groundbreaking research. Coming from the American environment and familiar with the power exercised by a dean, he had some difficulty in adjusting to being vice chancellor, when there were principals of three campuses who had a certain degree of autonomy. His was a major task in getting the institution as a whole to follow a single vision and subscribe to a strategic plan. Although frustrated on occasion by the difficulties of coordination, he never let it get the better of him and persisted in efforts to fashion a universally accepted vision and make a strategic plan meaningful for the institution as a whole. I do not believe that institutions like universities come easily to strategic planning. Academics almost naturally chafe at the discipline of the inherent reporting requirements. But to his credit, he persisted, and the notion and practice of strategic planning is one of his legacies.

One of his major achievements was the formation of the Open Campus, ending the notion of there being three major campuses in Jamaica, Barbados, and Trinidad and Tobago. Others were referred to by the pejorative term "non-campus countries". He championed indefatigably the notion of a regional tertiary education system as well as a regional accreditation system. Both of these have been frustrated in the bureaucracy of Caribbean politics, but that does not make them any less desirable and necessary. He was very focused on the Caribbean nature of the institution and making it the place of excellence to which all Caribbean people would turn for support. As a measure of his managerial skills and success, his 360 evaluation at the end of his first five-year contract, which was conducted by an external group of experienced evaluators, was rated as outstanding.

Our relations were excellent, and I could count on his keeping me abreast of the major developments and taking into account my advice and guidance when appropriate. His resignation after ten years was marked by a genuine outpouring of appreciation from all levels of the university, and there were numerous comments on his humility, his work ethic and his excellent interpersonal relations.

Hilary Beckles is an eminent historian with a powerful intellect who in his time as principal of the Cave Hill campus virtually transformed it both physically and academically. He was extraordinarily successful in establishing close links with the business community, leading to a mushrooming of new structures on campus, and his relationships with the government were parlayed into a steady increase in student numbers. He assumed the post of vice chancellor a year ago, and this short period has been marked by a series of brilliant initiatives focused on the creation of a more streamlined single institution and the projection of the university into the international arena.

While I refer to the vice chancellors specifically, I must also record my sincere appreciation for the dedication of the principals, pro-vice-chancellors and registrars, without exception most competent men and women, all committed to the excellence not only of their own particular campus or area of responsibility but patently to the maintenance of a first-rate regional institution.

During my term of office, I saw enrolment grow from fewer than twenty-three thousand students in 2002/2003 to about fifty thousand today. The Open Campus enrolment has remained steady at about five thousand students. The undergraduate body is predominantly female, with males predominating only in mechanical engineering. This predominance of female graduates is a global phenomenon, and there is no ready explanation. It cannot be healthy for society in the long term, but I have not encountered any satisfactory solution.

THE CEREMONIAL

Graduation ceremonies are a high point in the university's calendar, and at each of the forty-three graduation ceremonies, I have addressed some issue relevant to the university and tertiary education rather than simply reciting a list of university achievements. Having to prepare a different topic for each campus has been taxing, but judging by the feedback, it has been worthwhile.

On several occasions, I have referred to what I consider the essential roles of the modern university. Of course, there must be an unswerving commitment to excellence. There is the traditional credentialling role, as society needs institutions to certify certain levels of competence in citizens who perform the myriad duties essential for the functioning of our institutions. But in today's world, credentialling cannot be enough, as there

The Return of the Pelican: Back at the UWI

are several businesses which confine themselves to credentialling without undertaking the other major functions of universities. The most important function by far is the generation of information and its inculcation as knowledge into the young. There will always be a balance between the constitutive and the instrumental value of knowledge.

I often cautioned against the commodification of knowledge and the press of society's employers to have graduates who are "job ready". I argue, rather, that the emphasis in a university must be in producing graduates who are "job prepared", in the sense that they will be equipped to take on the myriad occupations which tomorrow's world will demand but which are not yet envisaged today. This form of preparation must involve inculcating the habit and practice of critical, logical thinking and attention to ethical practice. On more than one occasion I have warned that although the stress on innovation and entrepreneurship is a modern imperative, this must not be translated into undue obeisance to the disciplines of science, technology, engineering and mathematics and deprecation of the humanities. The theory of the triple helix of innovation has been attractive to me – emphasizing the interdependence of the university, business and the government. I have stressed that the university must have care for the mores and values of the society, embracing justice, truth and equity, and championing human rights. Our university must also tell the story of the Caribbean people.

I know that there is often controversy over the role of governments, especially since government financial contribution has declined over the years, but I hold that to the extent that tertiary education is a mix of public and private good, the cost must be shared between the government and the individual. I never fail to emphasize the importance of maintaining the regional nature of the university and contend that its physical dispersion is but another manifestation of the unending quest to perfect an institution to be optimally supportive of the aspirations of all Caribbean people.

I have always appealed to the graduates to be good alumni, as they are our ambassadors. They are urged to give back to their alma mater and to be good Pelicans – referring to the characteristic of the mythical bird that plucked its breast to feed its young. They might remember what Laertes says to Claudius:

THE GROOMING OF A CHANCELLOR

> To his good friends thus wide I'll ope my arms
> And, like the kind life-rendering pelican
> Repast them with my blood. . . .

I have persisted in greeting each graduate by name and shaking his or her hand. With the growth in the student population, this has meant an increase in annual graduation ceremonies from seven to thirteen, and over the years, I have greeted some seventy-five thousand graduates. There is frequent discussion as to whether this practice is the most efficient way of marking the formal graduation. However, student evaluations consistently prize individual attention, and it is important to them to be greeted by the chancellor. For many of them and their relatives, this represents a major occasion, as often they are the first graduate in the family. Clearly a balance will have to be found between operational efficiency and the symbolic value to the graduates and their relatives.

I also believe in the ritual of the graduation ceremonies. While I understand and encourage enthusiasm at a time when there is justifiable joy and exaltation, this should not mar the formal beauty of the occasion, which is a critical event in the lives of the graduands, their relatives and the institution.

The citations of the public orators have been a source of immense pleasure. The university has been fortunate in its choice of public orators, and I think there would be general agreement that in the past thirteen years the doyens of them all have been Eddie Baugh and Henry Fraser. They combined wit, elegance of phrase and clarity of diction with charming and perceptive explanations of the qualities that made the individual worth of an honorary degree. Of course, some honorary graduates bring with them the flamboyance of their professions. When the famous calypsonian Madam Rose was given her honorary degree, she sang one of her famous calypsos, then a second, and as she shook her hips and launched into another, there was mild consternation in the company.

The valedictorian addresses have been an interesting window into the thinking of the young and their appreciation of the institution. A remarkable feature of the majority has been the passionate defence of the regional nature of the university. They see this as perhaps more important than the knowledge they acquired and cite frequently their friendships across the Caribbean and similarities among them that they have come to appreciate. This always pleased me immensely. Even students in the Open Campus speak feelingly of their interaction across distance and cite geographic separation as being no barrier to developing the Caribbean or West Indian consciousness that they bear with pride.

Of course, there have been humorous aspects to some of our ceremonies. At a reception before one, a graduate said to me, "Chancellor, I shook your hand when I got my first degree. When I receive my master's degree tomorrow, may I hug you?" I demurred and said, "I would rather you did not, as I'm concerned about what you will suggest when you receive your PhD."

Epilogue

At the end of my final graduation ceremony at Mona in November 2016, I said that I had charted my own course in life – like Frank Sinatra, I had done it "my way". The memories around that song spark a segue into my lifelong interest in music. I had no musical talent at all, unfortunately, but that did not stop me from arguing over the relative merits of singers such as Sarah Vaughan and Ella Fitzgerald or various jazz artists. At Mona, I even wrote a jazz column for the *Pelican* magazine – creating a discography in which I included comments obtained from other aficionados on the merits of various artists. I found time for the jazz clubs in Kingston frequented by legendary musicians like trumpeter Sonny Bradshaw and trombonist Don Drummond. I admit that my love for music is linked to my love for dancing, and I amaze my colleagues now when I tell them that I once won a rock and roll contest at a medical association dance. My mother had taught me properly, insisting that if one perfected the Arthur Murray box step and had a sense of rhythm, one would be equipped for life. She was correct.

I think often of the conjunction of circumstances that allowed me to chart my own course, that allowed a little boy from a remote rural village in a small country to reach so far.

There was the teaching of Eileen and Clinton, the influence of the tight-knit family of seven, and the early inculcation of punctuality, truthfulness and respect for others. There was also the encouragement to logical expression and a commitment to excellence in everything I did. Competitiveness, discipline and optimism are personality traits which do not permit failure.

Next would have to be my good fortune in meeting my wife, Sylvan, indispensable to my adult life. I still marvel at how we fell in love in a time

Epilogue

and place in Jamaica when Chinese kept very much to themselves. I am not sure she was amused when at a medical alumni formal dinner, I spoke about the various stages of a man's life, maybe not with the profoundness of Shakespeare but I hope with more relevance. I said that the life of a man is divided into three stages, and it is critical that there be sequential harmony among them. In the first stage, when he is young and the hormones are raging, he needs a lover; in the more sedate middle years, he needs a friend; but in the autumn of his days, when the shadows lengthen and the leaves start to fall, he needs a nurse. I was fortunate in getting all three in one person. All the major decisions of our life together have been done in consultation, and I confess that some of the changes have been challenging for her, but with calm equanimity and boundless optimism, she would insist that everything would be all right. I reminded her recently of a comment of a student of mine, now in his middle years, that the secret of a successful life is in having "something interesting to leave home for and someone interesting to come home to". To which I would say a thankful *amen*. I must include my three children here – Carol, Andrew and Adrian – who have been a source of joy and pride to me and sometimes even a source of correction. Their paths to adulthood were not always smooth, but now that these have been traversed, I feel fortunate and privileged to count them as true and faithful friends.

I derived inspiration from a series of remarkable mentors. There was Harold Forde, the specialist physician with whom I worked when I returned to Barbados. Not only was he the essence of the "compleat physician" and an excellent teacher, but there was no equivocation over discipline and good medical care for his patients. His many kindnesses and concerns for my welfare and that of my family were remarkable.

There was Professor Max Rosenheim, later Lord Rosenheim, who took a paternal interest in Sylvan and me in London and whose counsel was invaluable, although he claimed he never gave advice.

John Waterlow, the doyen of mentors, was responsible not only for my scientific development but for my personal growth. I believe that more than anyone, he was responsible for demonstrating to me the value and worth of the Pygmalion effect. If someone believes in you and trusts you, you will feel a tremendous responsibility to reward that trust and perform well, often above your normal capabilities. John would lead by example; he would encourage but never scold. I recall only one occasion when John criticized me in public. I was scheduled to attend some scientific conference when I was in Boston, but I had to cancel because I had fallen ill with chicken pox. John was heard to remark in disgust, "That is damn foolishness. I expect my staff to have had such childhood illnesses before they come to work with me!" He believed firmly in the tradition of the scientific lineage. He could trace his own back through his physiology professor in Cambridge and several distinguished scientists, and he implied that he expected his scientific sons and daughters to do the same. I hope that some of my formers students think in this way of me.

I have few regrets. One which will always stay with me is that I was not at my mother's side when my father died. As the first child, I should have been there, and perhaps I was wrong to let financial considerations take precedence over filial responsibilities.

I regret not having been elected director general of WHO, not so much for personal reasons, but because it would have been a tremendous feat for my country and evidence that there is no special geographical distribution of talent.

I also regret that while there has been significant positive change, the progress in mobilizing our alumni to be a major force in the university has not been as rapid as I envisaged at the beginning of my term of office as chancellor. I trust that our Pelicans will sing more loudly in the future.

More than outweighing these, however, have been many incredible sources of satisfaction in my career. If I had to cite the most gratifying aspect, it would be the impact I have had on my students. I enjoyed, and still enjoy, teaching, and I continue to get a thrill when I transmit some concept to a student and see from the reaction that it has been grasped and internalized. Being a teacher has to be one of life's most satisfying callings.

I derived immense gratification from the privilege of being a personal care physician. In that profession, I got to see all the dimensions of what makes us human. There was the privilege of helping to heal, and there was the privilege of counselling and the profound satisfaction of relieving fear and doubt. There was satisfaction in accompanying a patient in the decision to adopt or reject a therapy and knowing the decision was born of trust. There was also the humbling experience of being faithful to the essential characteristics of good medicine – to prevent illness, to cure, to rehabilitate, and, when the time comes, to help another die with dignity. This last is often forgotten, as the technological imperative tends to see death as failure.

I have known the highs and lows of research – of establishing the correctness of a hypothesis but also, sometimes, of producing data to show that some cherished and carefully crafted thesis cannot be sustained. I have appreciated how humbling it is to make a small advance in scientific knowledge, only to have it open up many more questions that are beyond my technical capacity to answer. And, of course, one has to subject oneself to the scrutiny of one's peers. Yet overall, the camaraderie of my research colleagues is something I will always treasure.

I have had enduring pleasure from being part of and leading a team that cares for the public's health and is able to prevent disease in populations. There have been moments of high drama amid the routine that often marks such work: the dramatic appearance of cholera in the Americas after centuries of absence; the unfolding of the horrors of HIV/AIDS; moments of political tension and even wars. There has also been the enervating but chastening experience of visiting some remote village and observing firsthand the commitment of health workers to helping a fellow human being, travelling by mule, by bicycle or by boat to carry out essential life-saving duties.

The PAHO region was the first to eliminate poliomyelitis as the result of a magnificent campaign I described earlier. A committee was established to certify that the Americas was free of polio, and it reported its findings regarding this major public health achievement at a meeting in the PAHO council room to resounding applause. The occasion moved me tremendously. I recall saying emotionally and with shaking voice that through the applause I could hear the voices of the children of the Americas at play, rejoicing that never again would one of them have to walk with caliper or crutch because of polio.

Central America was in turmoil, and the PAHO director, Dr Macedo, had conceived the brilliant initiative of "Health as a Bridge for Peace", the idea being that health was a non-conflictive area around which men and women could find consensus and common cause and build a bridge for understanding. I visited El Salvador on an immunization day as part of the initiative. On that day, the guns were still – not a shot was fired. The government forces sent out their jeeps and advised people to come and have their children vaccinated, and the rebel forces did the same. One of my favourite photographs is of a soldier with an AK-47 slung over his shoulder helping to vaccinate a child.

I have experienced immense pride and satisfaction in being chancellor of my university – seeing it grow in numbers and influence, and knowing that I have done my best to continue the tradition of excellence set by my illustrious predecessors. Although as chancellor I did not have an executive role, I came to appreciate the more than symbolic nature of the office and that it contributes in some indefinable way to public appreciation of the institution. I am also satisfied that the decorum of the ritual of our ceremonies over the years has enhanced public appreciation of the institution.

I am content at this stage with my intellectual production. I sometimes review with modest satisfaction my two hundred publications in peer-reviewed journals, one hundred and eighty major lectures, speeches and named orations, fifty graduation addresses, and, in recent times, a dozen eulogies and tributes, together with books, book chapters, abstracts and numerous commentaries on a wide range of subjects. It gives me pleasure to know that my accumulated experience can be put to use through the various committees, commissions and reviews in which I participate, the lectures I give and the occasions when my advice is sought.

To date I have lived a full and I trust useful life and indeed travelled many highways, but nothing I have seen or heard has dimmed the feeling that was perhaps latent in my decision to study at a university in the West Indies. There are many aspects of Caribbean affairs about which I am passionate. I still retain a jealous pride in things Caribbean and a commitment to service to the Caribbean. I have a deep and abiding faith in the inevitability of acceptance of the power of functional cooperation for the betterment of our people. Perhaps *faith* is not the correct expression, as faith by definition is belief without data, and I have the data to show that my beliefs are not unfounded fantasy. There have been stumbles and hitches in some areas, but I believe in the inevitable progression towards

Epilogue

more closeness in the Caribbean and the strength of the instruments such as health and education to counteract and overcome the natural fissiparous tendencies of any grouping. I could cite as evidence the expressions of the valedictorians whom I have heard over the past thirteen years and who have moved me with their eloquent affirmations of commitment to Caribbean education and the regional idea and ideal. I can testify to the value of cooperation in health as well. I have seen the concrete demonstration of the contribution in these areas by our university, my university, which has not deviated from the injunction implied in the Declaration of Grand Anse by the CARICOM Heads of Government that it should be a regional institution indefinitely. Given the above and the frequent demonstration that our size is no measure of our talent or our ambition, I do not shrink from my optimism for our region.

I ended one of my last graduation addresses by bidding the graduates and the university farewell, and clarified that I did not intend it to suggest an irrevocable parting. I meant it in the pristine sense of "fare thee well", and I made that wish for their sakes and mine.

Farewell.

APPENDIX 1

Lectures and Formal Presentations

1979

Medical Research in the Caribbean (Dr Charles Duncan O'Neale Memorial Lecture, Queen Elizabeth Hospital), Bridgetown, Barbados, November.

1989

Health Arising from the West (Celebration of the Fortieth Anniversary of the University of the West Indies), Kingston, Jamaica, May.

1990

Environmental Health for All (Twenty-first Anniversary of the Barbados Sanitation Service Authority), Bridgetown, Barbados, September.

Health and Democracy (Parliamentary meeting), Kingston, Jamaica, October.

Health in the Caribbean and Latin America: Problems and Prospects (Barbados Independence Lecture), Toronto, Canada, November.

1991

Prevention: Goal for the 90s – Lessons to Be Learned for International Health (Society of Alumni Annual Reunion, Johns Hopkins University), Baltimore, Maryland, April.

Appendix 1: Lectures and Formal Presentations

Health and Tourism: The Intersectoral Linkages (Second Conference on International Travel Medicine), Atlanta, GA, May.

Alumni and Their University (First Awards Dinner of the UWI Guild of Graduates, Washington, DC Chapter), Washington, DC, June.

Tourism Health and the Environment (Tourism Health and the Environment Conference), Tobago, October.

Salud y Turismo (II Congreso Nacional de Turismo y Salud), Puerto Vallarta, Jalisco, Mexico, November.

Public Health for All (Sixth International Congress of the World Federation of Public Health Associations), Atlanta, GA, November.

1992

Caribbean Health and Health Research (Thirty-seventh Annual Commonwealth Caribbean Medical Research Council, International Trade Center), Curaçao, Netherland Antilles, April.

The Public Health and Development (Johns Hopkins University School of Hygiene and Public Health Convocation), Baltimore, Maryland, May.

Prospects and Challenges for the Health Sector (Annual Health Convention of Ministers of Health), Guyana, September.

Health in Housing: The Past, Present and Future (Conference on Health Housing in the Americas, State University of New York at Buffalo), Buffalo, New York, October.

Caribbean Health and Labour (Eleventh Triennial Caribbean Congress of Labour), Antigua, November.

Health and Tourism: A Philosophy for Its Development in the Americas (Inter-American Conference on Food Protection and Tourism), Cancun, Mexico, November.

1993

Sir Harry on Health in the Nineties (Sir Harry Annamunthodo Lecture), Kingston, Jamaica, May.

The Caribbean Health Promotion Charter (Caribbean Health Promotion Conference), Trinidad and Tobago, June.

Appendix 1: Lectures and Formal Presentations

The Health and Tourism Partners: Concepts, Roles and Prospects (Travel and Tourism Research Association Conference), British Columbia, Canada, June.

Environmental Health and Sustainable Tourism Development (Conference on Environmental Health and Tourism), Nassau, Bahamas, November.

On PAHO and Public Health (Fiftieth Anniversary Celebration, School of Public Health, University of California at Berkeley), Berkeley, California, November.

Capistrano in the Caribbean (Medical Alumni Association, University of the West Indies), Mona, November.

1994

Presencia de la Organización Panamericana de la Salud en la Salud Pública del Continente en el Siglo XX y Más Allá (Los 90 Años de la OPS y Primer Encuentro Iberoamericano de Historiadores de la Salud Pública), Havana, Cuba, February.

Health, the Indispensable Component (Workshop on Health and Environment in Sustainable Development, Barbados Community College), Barbados, April.

La Cooperación Técnica en las Americas (Conferencia "A Saude de Todos um Desafio para o Brasil, no Final do Seculo"), Brazil, June.

Images of our Health (Caribbean Media Awards for Excellence in Health and Journalism), Bridgetown, Barbados, September.

Election Address as Director of the Pan American Health Organization (Pan American Sanitary Conference), Washington, DC, September.

1995

Health in Our Time (Ceremony of Installation as Director of PAHO), Washington, DC, January.

The Kind of World We Live In (Forty-eighth Session of FICSA Council), Washington, DC, February.

A Healthy Press (Barbados Association of Journalists), Bridgetown, Barbados, March.

Health and the National Security (Distinguished Lecture Series, University of the West Indies), March.

Appendix 1: Lectures and Formal Presentations

Of Health and Heroes (Honour Award Banquet, the Gleaner Company), Kingston, Jamaica, March.

The Future of the Health System in Latin America and the Caribbean (Harvard International Health Leadership Forum), Boston, Massachusetts, June.

Health and Democracy (Permanent Council of the OAS), Washington, DC, September.

Faces of Health Reform (Second Canadian Conference of International Health), Ottawa, Canada, November.

The Context of Reform in the Caribbean (Extraordinary Meeting of the Caribbean Ministers Responsible for Health), Montego Bay, Jamaica, November.

The Primacy of Life Beyond All Human Conditions Everywhere on Health (Tenth International Conference of the Pontifical Council for Pastoral Assistance to Health Care Workers, "From Hippocrates to Good Samaritan"), Vatican City, November.

1996

The Profession, the Public and Health Reform (Trinidad and Tobago Medical Association), Port of Spain, Trinidad and Tobago, March.

Every Child Wanted Healthy, Educated, Safe and Loved (Children First: A Global Forum, hosted by the Carter Center and the Task Force for Child Survival and Development), Atlanta, Georgia, April.

La OPS de Ayer, Hoy y Mañana (Ministry of Health of Argentina), Buenos Aires, Argentina, April.

Cooperación Técnica de la OPS/OMS (Academia Nacional de Medicina), Santafé de Bogotá, Colombia, April.

Políticas de Salud y Salud Mental en América Latina y el Caribe (Reunión de evaluación de la iniciativa para la reestructuración de la atención psiquiátrica en América Latina), Panama City, Panama, June.

Beyond Medical Care: Policies for Health in the Next Century (Ninth Congress of the International Association of Health Policy), Montreal, Canada, June.

The House That John Built (Festschrift for Professor John C. Waterlow), London, England, June.

Appendix 1: Lectures and Formal Presentations

Old Challenges in New Skins (Fifteenth Meeting of the Conference of Ministers Responsible for Health), Port of Spain, Trinidad and Tobago, July.

Better Health in the Bahamas (Public lecture hosted by the UWI Medical Alumni Association), Nassau, Bahamas, September.

Salud y el Desarrollo Humano: El rol de los parlamentos (I Conferencia Panamericana de la Organización Internacional de Médicos Parlamentarios), Santa Cruz de la Sierra, Bolivia, October.

Health and Human Rights: The equity issue (Second International Conference on Health and Human Rights, Harvard University), Boston, Massachusetts, October.

1997

Infectious Diseases: A Global Problem (First International Underwriting Congress), Mexico City, Mexico, February.

La Equidad y la Salud: Una meta para todos (III Reunión del Consejo de Coordinación Internacional del INPPAZ), Buenos Aires, Argentina, March.

Global Health: The Paradigm, Policy and Program Implications (National Council for International Health Series, GWU Hospital), Washington, DC, August.

Bioética (Ceremonia de clausura del Curso de Magister en Bioética), Santiago de Chile, Chile, August.

Global Survival: A Convergence of Faith and Science (Fifth World Bank Conference on Environmental and Socially Sustainable Development), Washington, DC, October.

La Equidad y la Tecnología en Salud (Academia Nacional de Medicina), Rio de Janeiro, Brazil, November.

1998

Health for All: From Vision to Action (Symposium on National Strategy for Renewal of Health for All), Washington, DC, February.

Violence, Health and the Media (Inter-American Press Association), San Juan, Puerto Rico, March.

Health Information for All (Fourth Pan American Congress on Health Science Information), San José, Costa Rica, March.

Appendix 1: Lectures and Formal Presentations

Health Challenges for the Twenty-first Century: The Role of Institutions (Ministerial Roundtable on Health Challenges for the Twenty-first Century – II Summit of the Americas), Santiago, Chile, April.

The Cardiovascular Disease Pandemic (PAHO/NHLBI/FIC/WB Conference on Global Shifts in Disease Burden), Washington, DC, May.

Guarding the Public's Health (Eighty-ninth Annual Conference of the Canadian Public Health Association), Montreal, Canada, June.

La Cooperación Sanitaria Institucional (Jornadas de Cooperación Sanitaria, X Aniversario de la Agencia Española de Cooperación Internación y el 50avo. Aniversario de la OMS), Madrid, Spain, June.

Pride in the Product (Fiftieth Anniversary Celebration of the University of the West Indies), Kingston, Jamaica, July.

Hacia un Envejecimiento Sano (Reunión sobre el Mercado Común del Sur [MERCOSUR] y proyección Social. Adulto Mayor, Intercambio de Experiencias Regionales), Montevideo, Uruguay, September.

La Etica Biomédica (Ceremonia de la creación de la Comisión Nacional Biomédica), Buenos Aires, Argentina, September.

The Future of Medicine: Issues and Challenges (Fifth General Assembly of the World Medical Association), Ottawa, Canada, October.

Women, Wine and Song (Global Links), Pittsburgh, Pennsylvania, October.

Health and Human Development in the Global Economy (Seminar/Workshop on Health and Human Development in the New Global Economy: Experiences, Opportunities and Risks in the Americas, the University of Texas Medical Branch at Galveston), Galveston, Texas, October.

Reforma Sectorial y las Funciones Esenciales de Salud (II Conferencia Panamericana de Educación en Salud Pública), Mexico City, Mexico, November.

1999

The Interests of the Pan American Health Organization (Inauguration Ceremony of second term as Director of PAHO), Washington, DC, February.

La Salud y el Desarrollo Humano: Una perspectiva local (III Congreso Regional de las Américas sobre municipios y comunidades saludables), Medellín, Colombia, March.

Appendix 1: Lectures and Formal Presentations

PAHO and the Public's Health (Yale University), New Haven, Connecticut, June.

Health and Well Being (Hubert H. Humphrey Fellowship Program "Building a World Together: The Humphrey Legacy"), Washington, DC, June.

Universities and the Health of the Disadvantaged (Global Conference on Universities and the Health of the Disadvantaged: Building Coalitions with the Health Professions, Local Governments, and Their Communities, University of Arizona), Tucson, Arizona, July.

The Publishing Enterprise at the Pan American Health Organization (VI Meeting of WHO Interregional Committee on Policy and Coordination of Publications), Washington, DC, July.

Equity in Health (IX World Congress of Psychiatry), Hamburg, Germany, August.

Universidades Para un Mundo Más Sano (Universidad nacional mayor de San Marcos), Lima, Perú, August.

2000

La Salud en una Sociedad Mejor (Centro Interamericano de Estudios de Seguridad Social), Mexico, D.F., Mexico, March.

Equidad y Salud (Inauguración de la Biblioteca Virtual de Salud), Asunción, Paraguay, March.

Health and Quality of Life: Our Municipalities in an Era of Globalization (Third Conference of Local Health Authorities of the Americas), Quebec, Canada, March.

La Salud y el Desarrollo Económico en las Américas (X Jornadas Nacionales, IX Internacionales y I Congreso Americano de Economía de la Salud), Iguazú, Argentina, April.

Health and Development Revisited (Health Promotion Month), Port of Spain, Trinidad and Tobago, April.

Antimicrobial Resistance (Conference on Antimicrobial Resistance, jointly organized by the Royal Society of Medicine Foundation–Illinois, and The Royal Society of Medicine–London) Washington, DC, May.

Public Service in International Organizations (2000 Convocation for the Robert F. Wagner Graduate School of Public Service), New York, New York, May.

Appendix 1: Lectures and Formal Presentations

Health Promotion: Bridging the Equity Gap (Fifth Global Conference on Health Promotion), Mexico City, Mexico, June.

Pride in Our Health (Ministry of Health/UWI/PAHO/WHO), Bridgetown, Barbados, July.

Global Health Challenges (World Federation of Public Health Associations), Beijing, China, September.

El Futuro de la Salud Pública Veterinaria en las Américas (XVII Congreso Panamericano de Ciencias Veterinarias (XII PANVET), Panama City, Panama, September.

Health and the Quality of Life (Fourth Nursing Academic International Congress, George Mason University), Fairfax, Virginia, October.

Women's Health, the Double Burden (Memorial Lecture in Dedication to Dr Elizabeth Quamina), Port of Spain, Trinidad and Tobago, October.

La Salud Ambiental y las Grandes Metas de Nuestro Tiempo (Congreso de la Asociación Interamericana de Ingeniería Sanitaria y Ambiental-AIDIS), Porto Alegre, Brazil, December.

2001

Reply on the Conferment of the Order of the Caribbean Community (Twelfth Inter-Sessional Meeting of the Conference of Heads of Government of the Caribbean Community), Bridgetown, Barbados, February.

La Salud Pública al Comienzo del Milenio (IX Congreso Nacional de Investigación en Salud Pública), Cuernavaca, Morelos, Mexico, March.

Information: A Bridge Over the Divide (CRICS V Meeting, Knowledge for Change, Information and Knowledge for Health Equity), Havana, Cuba, April.

A Magnificent Obsession (Convocation address at Queen's University after receiving honorary degree of Doctor of Laws), Ontario, Canada, May.

The Way Forward (UWI Mona campus academic conference), Kingston, Jamaica, September.

Quality of Care in the New Generation of Health Sector Reform in the Americas (Eighteenth International Conference of the International Society for Quality in Health Care), Buenos Aires, Argentina, October.

La Equidad y el Futuro por Construir en el Campo de la Salud (Instituto de

Appendix 1: Lectures and Formal Presentations

Salud, Medio Ambiente, Economía y Sociedad), Buenos Aires, Argentina, October.

La Salud y la Reducción de la Pobreza: El papel del médico (Día de la medicina peruana), Lima, Perú, October.

The Shade of the Old Sandbox Tree (Old Harrisonian Society), St Michael, Barbados, November.

2002

Bread and Roses (Fifty-fifth Session of the FICSA Council Meeting), Washington, DC, February.

Promoting Health in the Twenty-first Century (Public address), Paramaribo, Suriname, February.

Equity and Health for All, Caracas, Venezuela, February.

La Estrategia de la Atención Primaria de Salud en la Búsqueda de la Equidad y el Desarrollo (Foro Nacional de Atención Primaria), Santo Domingo, República Dominicana, February.

Building a Bridge (Health and Environment Ministers of the Americas meeting), Ottawa, Canada.

Thanks and Praise (Sir Phillip Sherlock Award), Ocho Rios, Jamaica, March.

Partnering for Health (Forty-third Annual Meeting of Board of Governors of the Inter-American Development Bank), Fortaleza, Brazil, March.

The Future of International Technical Cooperation in Health (Celebration of the National Institute of Public Health), Cuernavaca, Mexico, March.

The Delay of Health and the Denial of Social Justice (Centro Interamericano de Estudios de Seguridad Social [CIESS]), Mexico City, Mexico, March.

Keeping the Faith (CARICOM Council on Human and Social Development), Georgetown, Guyana, April.

Los Desafíos en la Salud para *homo informaticus* (Ceremonia de conmemoración de los 25 años de BIREME), San Paulo, Brazil, April.

One Hundred Years of Solidarity (International Convention of Public Health, Centennial Session), Havana, Cuba, May.

Cooperation in Health and Agriculture (Seventieth General Session of the International Office of Epizooties), Paris, France, May.

Appendix 1: Lectures and Formal Presentations

Advancing to Our Past (Fortieth Anniversary of the Advisory Committee on Health Research [ACHR]), Washington, DC, June.

Formación de Alianzas en Pro de la Promoción de la Salud (Foro de Promoción de la Salud en las Américas y II Congreso Chileno de Promoción de la Salud, Promoción de la Salud: Empoderando y formando alianzas para la salud), Santiago, Chile, October.

Another Golden Age for Environmental Health (Inter-American Association of Sanitary and Environmental Engineering), Cancún, Mexico, October.

A Vision for Caribbean Health (University of the West Indies), Bridgetown, Barbados, November.

2003

Thanks for the Memories (World Health Organization's 111th Session of the Executive Board Meeting), Geneva, Switzerland, January.

No Sadness of Farewell (Final PAHO General Staff Meeting), Washington, DC, January.

1952 and All That (Fiftieth Anniversary of the University Hospital of the West Indies), Kingston, Jamaica, April.

The Prospect for Health and Wealth in the Caribbean (William Demas Memorial Lecture), Basseterre, St Kitts and Nevis, May.

Of Wilson and Wernicke (First Jeffrey Wilson Memorial Lecture, Association of Consultant Physicians of Jamaica), Kingston, Jamaica, September.

Education a Key Partner in a Multisectoral Response to HIV/AIDS (Conference on "HIV/AIDS: The Power of Education" sponsored by UNICA/UWI/UNESCO), Port of Spain, Trinidad and Tobago, October.

The Sanitary and Social Measures (ISSA Regional Conference for the Americas), St Michael, Barbados, November.

Globalization and the Challenges to Caribbean Health (Michael Manley Memorial Lecture), Kingston, Jamaica, December.

Voices of the Pelican (Installation address as Chancellor of the University of the West Indies), Bridgetown, Barbados, December.

Appendix 1: Lectures and Formal Presentations

2004

The Butchers, the Bakers, the Candlestick Makers (Commemoration Day, UWI), Kingston, Jamaica, February.

HIV/AIDS: Challenges to the Caribbean (Eighteenth Dr Eric Williams Memorial Lecture), Port of Spain, Trinidad and Tobago, June.

Public Good and Personal Gain: The Higher Education (Mona Academic Conference), Kingston, Jamaica, August.

Primary Health Care: 1978 and All That (Twenty-fifth Celebration of Alma Ata Declaration on Primary Health Care), Port of Spain, Trinidad and Tobago, September.

Stigma and Discrimination against HIV/AIDS: Challenges in the Caribbean (CARICOM-UK Champions for Change conference: Reduce Stigma and Discrimination against People Living with HIV/AIDS), St Kitts and Nevis, November.

2005

Social Capital, Ethics and Development: The Relevance for Health in Small States ("Ethics and Development Day", Inter-American Development Bank), Washington, DC, January.

Philanthropy in Developing Nations: Gifts and Giving in the Caribbean (Regional Conference of Relevance of Philanthropy in Developing Nations), Kingston, Jamaica, February.

Research Ethics: Hippocrates, Helsinki and Beyond (Research Ethics Conference at the University of the West Indies), Kingston, Jamaica, April.

For the Good of the Public's Health (General Meeting of the Barbados Association of Medical Practitioners), Bridgetown, Barbados, May.

Publish or Perish: The Case of HIV/AIDS (International Forum of the Caribbean Publishers Network), Montego Bay, Jamaica, May.

Mobilizing Political Will (Helsinki Conference), Helsinki, September.

Health for Development in the Americas (Organization of American States Lecture Series of the Americas), Washington, DC, October.

Immunization for All: A Condition for Health and Development (2005 Sabin Vaccine Institute Policy Colloquium), New York, New York, October.

Appendix 1: Lectures and Formal Presentations

Risk, Reward and Responsibility in the Land of Make-Believe (Caribbean Actuarial Association's Fifteenth Annual Conference), Montego Bay, Jamaica, December.

All for One and One for All: The University of the West Indies (Launch of the UWI Alumni Association), St Kitts and Nevis, December.

2006

HIV in the Caribbean: Importance of Awareness and Stigma for People and Populations (Caribbean Broadcast Media Leaders Summit on HIV/AIDS), Bridgetown, Barbados, May.

Convocation Address (Convocation for the Faculty of Agricultural and Environmental Sciences, McGill University and conferment of honorary degree Doctor of Science – Honoris Causa), Montreal, Canada, June.

Sexual and Reproductive Health in the Search for Development (Fiftieth Anniversary Meeting of the Family Planning Association of Trinidad and Tobago), Port of Spain, Trinidad and Tobago, June.

Increasing the Range of Human Choice: The Case for Health (Eleventh Sir Arthur Lewis Memorial Lecture), St Kitts, November.

The Fiftieth Stride: A Tale of Runnings at Mona (TMRU Fiftieth Anniversary Celebration), Kingston, Jamaica, November.

Accelerating Project Implementation in HIV/AIDS in the Caribbean (World Bank's Caribbean HIV/AIDS Projects Implementation and Training Workshop), St Lucia, December.

2007

Economics and HIV/AIDS in the Caribbean (2007 Caribbean Region Summit on HIV/AIDS), St Croix, US Virgin Islands, January.

El Costo de la Oportunidad, las Repercusiones en la Toma de Decisiones (Conferencia el costo de la oportunidad, repercusiones en la toma de decisiones), Santafé de Bogotá, Colombia, February.

Cooperating for Success in Health (Fifth Olive Trotman Memorial Lecture, Thirty-seventh Anniversary of the Barbados Public Workers' Co-operative Credit Union, Limited), St Michael, Barbados, May.

Appendix 1: Lectures and Formal Presentations

Dentistry in Paradise (Caribbean Dental Programme's Fifth Annual Convention), St Michael, Barbados, May.

The Case for a Policy and Practice of "Inclusion" (Barbados Evangelical Association Sub-Regional Faith-Based Forum Focusing on Inclusion and Human Sexuality in the Context of HIV and AIDS), Christ Church, Barbados, June.

2008

Thanks for the "First Sixty" (Commemorative service to mark the sixtieth anniversary of the University of the West Indies), Washington, DC, June.

Extending the Art of Medicine (First Eric Cruickshank Distinguished Lecture), Kingston, Jamaica, July.

Mirror, Mirror on the Wall (UWI Medical Alumni Association Banquet), Ocho Rios, Jamaica, July.

Peace, Pandemics and Pluralism (Caribbean Chronic Disease Conference, Inter-American Heart Foundation Science of Peace Award and Lecture), Bridgetown, Barbados, October.

Reflections on Some Ethical Issues Raised by HIV (Guyana National Faith-and-HIV Conference, UNAIDS), Georgetown, Guyana, December.

2009

The Many Faces of Health (Duke University School of Nursing, Office of Global and Community Health Initiatives), Durham, North Carolina, January.

Fields Beloved in Vain (Annual Dinner of Taylor Hall, UWI, Mona campus), Mona, Kingston, Jamaica, January.

You Can Get It If You Really Want (2009 Presidential Dinner, Society of Black Academic Surgeons), Seattle, Washington, April.

Of Robes and Roles in Medicine (Recognition of Graduates and Oath Taking Ceremony of the 2009 graduating class of the UWI School of Clinical Medicine and Research), Nassau, the Bahamas, June.

The Learned and Grave in Medicine (Annual Symposium and Banquet of the Association of Consultant Physicians of Jamaica), Kingston, Jamaica, September.

Wisdom, Wellness and Wealth (2009 Dr Bernard A. Sorhaindo Memorial Lecture), Roseau, Dominica, September.

Appendix 1: Lectures and Formal Presentations

2010

The Price of Privilege (School of Arts and Sciences and Graduate Studies Programme at Graduation Ceremony), St George's, Grenada, May.

The Highest Standards (2010 Symposium of the Medical Association of Jamaica), Kingston, Jamaica, June.

Of Alumni as We Are and Memories of the Way We Were (Tenth International Scientific and Reunion Conference of the UWI Medical Alumni Association), Bridgetown, Barbados, November.

2011

Cultivating Caribbean Cultural Regionalism (Inaugural Rex Nettleford Lecture), Kingston, Jamaica, February.

Of Pipettes and Pelicans and What Merris Saw (Ceremony to honour Professor John Waterlow), London, England, April.

Promoting and Protecting Your (Global) Health (FDA commissioner's Global Health Lectureship), Washington, DC, June.

Preparing the End of the Beginning for NCDs (Sir Gustav Nossal Global Health Oration), Melbourne, Australia, August.

Health Degendered Is Health Denied (Institute for Gender and Development Studies), UWI Cave Hill, St Augustine and Mona campuses, October–November.

2012

From NCD Declarations to Action (CAREM 2012: Transforming NCD Declarations to Actions), Brasilia, Brazil, May.

Next Generation Living (Rio-20 UN conference on sustainable development), Rio de Janeiro, Brazil, June.

Whence and Whither Caribbean Health in This Fiftieth Year (Sir Arthur Lewis Lecture, Sir Arthur Lewis Institute of Social and Economic Studies Conference, Fifty-Fifty: Critical Reflections in a Time of Uncertainty), Kingston, Jamaica, August.

Global Health Challenges and Opportunities (International Federation of Pharmaceutical Manufacturers and Associations Assembly). Geneva, Switzerland, October.

Appendix 1: Lectures and Formal Presentations

2013

Cave Hill Anniversary (Fiftieth anniversary of the establishment of the Cave Hill campus), Cave Hill, Barbados, February.

Tertiary Education in Evolution (Tenth Annual Dr Alister Francis Memorial Lecture), St John's, Antigua and Barbuda, February.

A Social Contract: Innovation in Health Professional Education for Establishing Trans-disciplinary Professionalism for Health (Global Forum workshop "Establishing Trans-disciplinary Professionalism for Health"), Washington, DC, May.

Emancipation: The Lessons and the Legacy – Emancipation and Health (Emancipation Lecture 2013), Kingston, Jamaica, July.

Science in Diplomacy: Can Evidence Trump Interests (Graduate Institute High-level Symposium "Health Diplomacy Meets Science Diplomacy"), Geneva, Switzerland, November.

Global Health in Universities (Emory Global Health Institute Distinguished Lecturer Series, Emory University), Atlanta, Georgia, November.

The Caribbean and Chronic Disease (Strengthening Health Systems, Supporting NCD Action: Advocating for Policies and Action), Port of Spain, Trinidad and Tobago, November.

The Role of Civil Society in the Prevention and Control of Noncommunicable Diseases (WHO European Ministerial Conference on the Prevention and Control of Noncommunicable Diseases in the Context of Health 2020), Ashgabat, Turkmenistan, December.

2014

Health Diplomacy, Science Diplomacy: Can the Twain Meet? (Institute of International Relations, University of the West Indies, St Augustine campus), St Augustine, Trinidad and Tobago, March.

Frank Worrell: Of Legends and Leaders (Frank Worrell Memorial Lecture, University of the West Indies, St Augustine campus), St Augustine, Trinidad and Tobago, May.

The Barbados Family Planning Association: Its Right to Exist (Fifty-ninth Annual General Meeting of the Barbados Family Planning Association), St Michael, Barbados, May.

Appendix 1: Lectures and Formal Presentations

Caribbean Accreditation Authority for Education in Medicine and Other Health Professions (Tenth Anniversary Conference of the Caribbean Accreditation Authority for Education in Medicine and Other Health Professions), Montego Bay, Jamaica, July.

Go Well! Go Red! (Trinidad and Tobago Heart Foundation's Fundraising Dinner and Red Dress Ball), Port of Spain, Trinidad and Tobago, November.

Reflections on the Book *Glimpses of a Global Life* (Launch of the memoirs of Sir Shridath Ramphal), OAS, Washington, DC, November.

2015

Health in All Policies: Control and Prevention of Chronic Noncommunicable Diseases (Sixteenth Public Health Research Congress), Cuernavaca, Morelos, Mexico, March.

Palliative Care: Raising Awareness through Collaboration, Education and Practice (Caribbean Region Palliative Care Conference 2015 "Raising Awareness through Collaboration, Education and Practice"), Kingston, Jamaica, April.

Of NCD's and Sounding the Horn of Health and Well-being (Opening Ceremony of the Golden Jubilee Symposium of the Medical Association of Jamaica) Kingston, Jamaica, June.

2016

Of Arms, the Hero and Demographics (Errol Barrow Memorial Lecture delivered during the sixty-second anniversary of the Democratic Labour Party), Bridgetown, Barbados, April.

Everything Is Going Your Way (Convocation address, graduation ceremony of the George Mason University College of Health and Human Services), Fairfax, Virginia, May.

Equity and Global Health (Gulbenkian 2016 Summer Course on Global Health and Health Diplomacy), Lisbon, Portugal, June.

The Quest for the Public's Health (Conference on the History of Public Health and Society in Latin America and the Caribbean), Port of Spain, Trinidad and Tobago, July.

The Compleat Physician (2016 Rolf Richards Distinguished Lecture), Kingston, Jamaica, September.

Appendix 1: Lectures and Formal Presentations

Implementing Sound Health Policies: The Case of NCDs in the Caribbean (Tenth Annual Research Day of the University of the West Indies School of Clinical Medicine and Research), Nassau, Bahamas, September.

Craftsmen of Our Fate: The Social Instruments of Our Craft (University of the West Indies' public lecture series, marking Barbados's fiftieth anniversary of independence), Cave Hill, Barbados, October.

The Role of the University in the National and Regional Communities (University of the Bahamas), Nassau, Bahamas, November.

APPENDIX 2

The University of the West Indies Graduation Addresses

Honouring the Tradition, Cave Hill, October 2003.

Removing the Barriers of Functional Unity, St Augustine, October 2003.

The Light Has Risen, Mona, November 2003.

The Imperative of Response to Natural Disasters, Cave Hill, October 2004.

A Disaster Resistant University, St Augustine, October 2004.

Pride in Our Brand, Mona, November 2004.

A University for All, Cave Hill, October 2005.

The University of the West Indies and the Knowledge Business, St Augustine, October 2005.

Chimes of the Bell, Mona, November 2005.

Chaguaramas and the Pelican, Cave Hill, October 2006.

The University and its Nations, St Augustine, November 2006.

Ours to Nourish: Alumni and the University, Mona, November 2006.

Will Everything Be Alright? St Augustine, November 2006.

Academic Alternatives, Cave Hill, October 2007.

Multiversity, Diversity: Are They Relevant to Our University? St Augustine, November 2007.

Public Understanding of the University, Mona, November 2007.

Appendix 2: The University of the West Indies Graduation Addresses

The Sixtieth Year, Cave Hill, October 2008.

Knowledge for Development: Caribbean Impact, Global Reach, St Augustine, October 2008.

The Gift of Reason, Mona, November 2008.

No End to Beginnings, Open Campus, inaugural graduation ceremony, St Lucia, October 2009.

Our Competitive Advantage, Cave Hill, October 2009.

Our Challenges, Our Opportunities and Our Responses, St Augustine, October 2009.

The University of the West Indies: Symbol or Instrument of Regionalism, Mona, November 2009.

Geography, Destiny and the University of the West Indies, Open Campus, St George's, Grenada, October 2010.

Strengthening the Bond: The West Indian Bond, Cave Hill, October 2010.

Celebrating our Jubilee, St Augustine, October 2010.

Confronting Crisis, Grasping Opportunity at Mona, November 2010.

The Fourth Child, Open Campus, Antigua and Barbuda, October 2011.

Growing with Confidence, St Augustine, October 2011.

Supporting National and Regional Development, Cave Hill, October 2011.

On Being a Good Steward, Mona, November 2011.

Of Poincianas and Pelicans, Open Campus, St Kitts and Nevis, October 2012.

Remembering Sir Carlisle Burton, Cave Hill, October 2012.

Celebrating the Fiftieth, St Augustine, October 2012.

The Many Faces of Our Academy, Mona, November 2012.

Educational Entrepreneurship, Open Campus, Grenada, October 2013.

The Faith of Our Founders in This Jubilee Year, Cave Hill, October 2013.

A University Partnering for Science and Technology, St Augustine, October 2013.

Sustaining the Enterprise, Mona, November 2013.

Celebrating Steady Growth, Open Campus, St Lucia, October 2014.

Encouraging Public Debate, Cave Hill, October 2014.

Appendix 2: The University of the West Indies Graduation Addresses

Sustaining Our Human Development, St Augustine, October 2014.

The University of the West Indies: A Resilient University, Mona, October 2014.

Our Rituals and Our Values, Open Campus, Antigua and Barbuda, October 2015.

The University and the Public's Health, Cave Hill, October 2015.

It Takes Many Disciplines, St Augustine, October 2015.

Making Our Mark, Mona, October 2015.

Fifty Years of Support, Cave Hill, October 2016.

The Times Are a-Changing, St Augustine, October 2016.

In This Great Future, Mona, October 2016.

Notes

CHAPTER 1

1. Ralph A. Jemmott, *A History of Harrison College: A Study of an Elite Educational Institution in a Colonial Polity* (N.p.: Ralph A. Jemmott, 2006).

CHAPTER 2

1. For a history of the University of the West Indies, see Philip Sherlock and Rex Nettleford, *The University of the West Indies: A Caribbean Response to the Challenge of Change* (London: Macmillan, 1990).
2. Aristotle, *The Nicomachean Ethics*, trans. David Ross; rev. with intro. and notes by Lesley Brown (London: Oxford University Press, 2009).
3. Francis Fukuyama, *The End of History and the Last Man* (New York: Free Press, 1992).
4. Martin Luther King, "1963 Letter from a Birmingam Jail", in *I Have a Dream. Writings and Speeches that Changed the World*, ed. James Melvin Washington (San Francisco: Harper, 1992).
5. D. Ashley and R. Bernal, "A Review of the Poliomyelitis Epidemics in Jamaica. The Immunization Policies and Socioeconomic Implications", *Disasters* 9 (1985): 139–43.
6. "On This Day in Jamaican History: Kendal Railway Tragedy", *Jamaica Magazine*, jamaicans.com/on-this-day-in-jamaican-history-kendal-railway-tragedy.
7. John S.R. Golding, *Ascent to Mona as Illustrated by a Short History of Jamaican Medical Care* (Kingston: Canoe Press, 1994), 63.
8. F.H. Shaw, S.E. Simon et al., "Barbiturate Antagonism", *Nature* 174 (1954): 402–3.

CHAPTER 3

1. Gaius Valerius Catullus, Carmen 46. Available at http://rudy.negenborn.net/catullus/text2/e46.htm.
2. A.L. Cochrane, *Effectiveness and Efficiency. Random Reflections on Health Service* (London: Nuffield Provincial Hospitals Trust, 1972).

CHAPTER 4

1. Terrence Forrester, David Picou and Susan Walker, *The Tropical Metabolism Research Unit, the University of the West Indies, Jamaica, 1956–2006: The House That John Built* (Kingston: Ian Randle, 2007). This constitutes a fiftieth anniversary history of the TMRU, including an account of its origin by John Waterlow.
2. G.A.O. Alleyne, "Renal and Cardiac Function in Severely Malnourished Jamaican Children", (MD thesis, London University, 1965).
3. B. Magee, *Popper* (London: Fontana/Collins, 1973). This is a synthesis of much of Popper's work.
4. P.B. Medawar, *Advice to a Young Scientist* (New York: Harper and Row, 1979).
5. P.B. Medawar, *The Art of the Soluble* (London: Methuen, 1967).
6. R.F. Pitts, "Renal Production and Excretion of Ammonia", *American Journal of Medicine* 36 (1964): 720–42.
7. A.D. Goodman, R.C. Fuisz et al., "Renal Gluconeogenesis in Acidosis, Alkalosis and Potassium Deficiency: Its Possible Role in Regulation of Renal Ammonia Production", *Journal of Clinical Investigation* 45 (1966): 612–19.
8. G.A.O. Alleyne, "Concentrations of Metabolic Intermediates in the Kidneys of Rats with Metabolic Acidosis", *Nature* 217 (1968): 847–48; G.A.O. Alleyne and G.H. Scullard, "Renal Metabolic Response to Acid Base Changes 1: Enzymatic Control of Ammoniagenesis in the Rat", *Journal of Clinical Investigation* 48 (1970): 364–70.
9. A list of publications from our group on this topic can be found in publication compendia such as ResearchGate.
10. G.A. Alleyne, "Medical Research in the Caribbean" (Charles Duncan O'Neale Memorial Lecture, Queen Elizabeth Hospital, Bridgetown, Barbados, 16 November 1979), in *Health and Development in Our Time: Selected Speeches of Sir George Alleyne*, ed. Henry Fraser (Kingston: Ian Randle, 2008), .

11. G. Giglioli, *Malarial Nephritis* (London: J. & A. Churchill, 1932), 16.
12. G. Giglioli, *Demerara Doctor: An Early Success against Malaria – The Autobiography of a Self-taught Physician, 1897–1975*, ed. Chris Curtis; foreword by Chris Curtis (London: Smith-Gordon, 2006).

CHAPTER 5

1. "Proposal for the Participation of Project Hope in Graduate Medical Education Programme at the University of the West Indies", Faculty of Medicine FMP 53, amended 1970/71; R.C. Morrow and R. Carpente, *Project Hope and the Training of Specialists in the West Indies* (Millwood, VA: Project HOPE Health Sciences Education Center, 1980).
2. Agreement concerning initiation of postgraduate training programmes in Medical Education (personal copy).
3. "Report on Visit of a Working Party to Universities in Ghana, Nigeria and Sierra Leone, January/February 1973" (Commonwealth Foundation, Occasional Paper no. 20, Universities of the West Indies and of Guyana).
4. H. Ho Ping Kong, with Michael Posner, *The Art of Medicine: Healing and the Limits of Technology* (Toronto: ECW Press, 2014).

CHAPTER 6

1. M. Cueto, *The Value of Health: A History of the Pan American Health Organization* (Rochester, NY: Rochester University Press, 2007); PAHO, *Pro Salute Novi Mundi: A History of the Pan American Health Organization* (Washington, DC: PAHO, 1992); G.A.O. Alleyne, "The Pan American Health Organization's First 100 Years: Reflections of the Director", *American Journal of Public Health* 92 (2002): 1890–93.
2. J. Duffy, *Ventures in World Health: The Memoirs of Fred Lowe Soper*, Scientific Publication no. 355 (Washington, DC: PAHO, 1977).
3. C.A. De Quadros, J.K. Andrus, J.M. Olive, et al., "Eradication of Poliomyelitis in the Americas", *Pediatric Infectious Disease Journal* 10 (1991): 222–29.
4. G.A.O. Alleyne, F. Luelmo, R. Plaut and G. Schmunis, *Acute Respiratory Infections in Children*, Scientific Publication no. 493 (Washington, DC: PAHO, 1983).

5. G.A. Alleyne and H.C. Dyer, "Cooperation in Health in the Commonwealth Caribbean", *Caribbean Affairs* 3 (1990): 135–50.
6. G.A.O. Alleyne and Kareb A. Sealey, "Whither Caribbean Health: A Study", Occasional Paper no. 5 (West Indian Commission Secretariat, 1992).
7. See the communiqué issued at conclusion of Twenty-fifth Conference of the CARICOM Heads of Government, and the CARPHA website for a description of its organization and functions: http://caricom.org/media-center/communications/communiques/communique-issued-at-the-conclusion-of-the-twenty-first-inter-sessional-meeting and http://carpha.org.

CHAPTER 7

1. M. Hammer and J. Champy, *Reengineering the Corporation* (New York: Harper Business, 1993); R.L. Manganelli and M.M. Klein, *The Reengineering Handbook. A Step-by-Step to Business Transformation* (New York: AMACOM, 1994).

CHAPTER 8

1. J.B. Lockey, *Essays in Pan-Americanism* (Port Washington, NY: Kennikat Press, 1939).
2. T.S. Eliot, *The Rock* (New York: Harcourt Brace, 1934), 7.
3. H. Cleveland, *The Knowledge Executive; Leadership in an Information Society* (New York: Truman Talley Books/E.P. Dutton, 1985).
4. *The Yellow Emperor's Classic of Internal Medicine*, trans. Ilza Veith (Berkeley: University of California, 1975).
5. P.M. Blau, *Bureaucracy in Modern Society* (New York: Random House, 1968).
6. P.F. Drucker, *The Concept of the Corporation* (New York: Mentor Executive Library, 1946). This was the first book by Drucker that I read in about 1975, and subsequently I followed his publications avidly, until I became disenchanted with his *The Leader of the Future*.
7. G.A.O. Alleyne, "Towards a Taxonomy of Technical Cooperation in Health", *Bulletin of the Pan American Health Organization* 25 (1991): 356–66.
8. UNDP, "The Buenos Aires Plan of Action for Promoting and Implementing Technical Cooperation among Developing Countries" (UNDP, 1978), http://ssc.undp.org/content/dam/ssc/documents/Key%20Policy%20Documents/BAPA.pdf.9.

9. "The Kuwait Declaration on Technical Cooperation amongst Developing Countries/Déclaration de Koweit sur la Coopération Technique parmi les Nations En Développement." *Africa Development/Afrique et Développement* 2, no. 2 (1977): 125–33. http://www.jstor.org/stable/24486365.
10. PAHO, "International Technical Cooperation in Health" (PAHO/AD/94.1, 1994).
11. G.A.O. Alleyne and J.M. Sotelo, "Technical Cooperation among Countries in the Americas" (internal PAHO document prepared for the interregional consultation on TCC programming in health, Jakarta, Indonesia, 1993).
12. G.A.O. Alleyne, "Technical Cooperation in the World Health Organization" (internal PAHO document prepared for the interregional consultation on TCC programming in health, Jakarta, Indonesia, 1993).
13. PAHO, "Technical Cooperation among Countries: Pan Americanism in the Twenty-first Century" (CSP25/9, 1998).
14. M. Gould, "Strategic Control in the Decentralized Firm", *Sloan Management Review* (Winter 1991): 69–81.
15. C. Weiss, *Evaluation Research: Methods for Assessing Program Effectiveness* (Englewood Cliffs, NJ: Prentice Hall, 1972).

CHAPTER 10

1. J.C. Collins and J.I. Porras, *Built to Last: Successful Habits of Visionary Companies* (New York: Harper Business, 1994).
2. PAHO, *Public Health in the Americas: Conceptual Renewal, Performance Assessment and Bases for Action*, Scientific Publication no. 589 (Washington, DC: PAHO, 2002).
3. PAHO, *The Crisis of Public Health: Reflections for the Debate*, Scientific Publication no. 540 (Washington, DC: PAHO, 1992).

CHAPTER 11

1. UNAIDS, CARICOM, "A Study of the Pan Caribbean Partnership against HIV/AIDS (PANCAP) Common Goals, Shared Responsibilities" (UNAIDS Best Practice Collection, 2004).
2. http://documents.worldbank.org/curated/en/379611468010840800/World-Bank-financed-HIV-projects-in-the-Caribbean-lessons-for-working-with-small-states-an-after-action-review-of-HIV-projects-financed-by-the-World-Bank-in-the-Caribbean.

3. George A.O. Alleyne and Rose-Marie Belle-Antione, *HIV and Human Rights: Legal and Policy Perspectives on HIV and Human Rights in the Caribbean* (Kingston: University of the West Indies Press, 2013).
4. M. Ul Haq, *Reflections on Human Development* (New York: Oxford University Press, 1995); UNDP, *Human Development Report* (Oxford: Oxford University Press, 1990).
5. G. Alleyne, "Health and Economic Growth: Policy Reports and the Making of Policy", in *Health and Growth*, ed. M. Spence and M. Lewis (Washington, DC: Commission on Growth and Development, World Bank, 2009).
6. G. Alleyne, A. Binagwaho, A. Haines et al., "Embedding Non-communicable Diseases in the Post-2015 Development Agenda", *Lancet* 381 (2013): 566–74.
7. Jeffrey Sachs, "Macroeconomics and Health: Investing in Health for Economic Development. Report of the Commission on Macroeconomics and Health", World Health Organization, Geneva, 2001.
8. PAHO, CARICOM Secretariat, *Report of the Caribbean Commission on Health and Development* (Kingston: Ian Randle, 2006).
9. S.J. Hoffman, "The Evolution, Etiology and Eventualities of the Global Health Security Regime", *Health Policy and Planning* 25 (2010): 501–22.
10. Ibid.
11. R. Fisher R and W. Ury, *Getting to Yes: Negotiating Agreement without Giving In* (London: Penguin, 1991).

Selected Bibliography

Alleyne, G.A.O. *Health and Development in Our Time: Selected Speeches of Sir George Alleyne*, edited by Henry Fraser. Kingston: Ian Randle, 2008.

———. *A Quest for Equity/En busca de la equidad: Selected Speeches*. Washington, DC: PAHO 2002.

———. "Renal and Cardiac Function in Severely Malnourished Jamaican Children". MD thesis, London University, 1965.

Alleyne, George A.O., and Rose-Marie Belle-Antione. *HIV and Human Rights: Legal and Policy Perspectives on HIV and Human Rights in the Caribbean*. Kingston: University of the West Indies Press, 2013.

Alleyne, G.A.O., and D. Cohen. "Health, Economic Growth, and Poverty Reduction". Report of Working Group 1 of the Commission on Macroeconomics and Health. World Health Organization, Geneva, 2002.

Alleyne, G.A.O., A. Hay, D. Picou, J.P. Stanfield and R.G. Whitehead. *Protein Energy Malnutrition*. London: Edward Arnold, 1976.

Alleyne, G.A.O., and Karen A. Sealey. "Whither Caribbean Health: A Study". Occasional Paper no. 5. West Indian Commission Secretariat, 1992.

Forrester, Terrence, David Picou and Susan Walker. *The Tropical Metabolism Research Unit, the University of the West Indies, Jamaica, 1956–2006: The House That John Built*. Kingston: Ian Randle, 2007.

Golding, John S.R. *Ascent to Mona as Illustrated by a Short History of Jamaican Medical Care*. Kingston: Canoe Press, 1994.

Jamison, D.T., J.G. Brenan, A.R Measham, G. Alleyne, M. Claeson, D.B. Evans, P. Jha, A. Mills and P. Musgrove, eds. *Disease Control Priorities in Developing Countries*. 2nd ed. Washington, DC: Oxford University Press and the World Bank, 2006.

PAHO, CARICOM Secretariat. *Report of the Caribbean Commission on Health and Development*. Kingston: Ian Randle, 2006.

Sherlock, Philip, and Rex Nettleford. *The University of the West Indies: A Caribbean Response to the Challenge of Change*. London: Macmillan, 1990.

Index

Page numbers in italics refer to photographs.

Abbadabba, Otto, 158
Acuna, Dr Hector, 97, 99, 100, 122, 125, 126, 127; and GA as PAHO director, 128; on PAHO and the Caribbean, 106–7
Addams, Jane, 78–79
Adonijah, 8
Advice to a Young Scientist (Medawar), 66, 67
African universities, linkages with, 86–87
Aiken, Denis, 171
Aiston, Ed, 121
Alcoa Foundation, 91
Ali, Muhammad, 91
Alice of Athlone, Princess, 57
Allenbury Prize, 38
Alleyne, Adrian (son), 61, 93, *180*, 225
Alleyne, Andrew (son), 61, 93, *180*, 225
Alleyne, Carol (daughter), 61, 76, 93, *180*, 225
Alleyne, Cecily (sister), 8, *177*
Alleyne, Clinton Ogarren (father), 1–2, 10–11, 12, 19, 53, 224
Alleyne, Cynthia (sister), 2, 5–6, 13, 14, 50–51, 55, 121, *177*
Alleyne, Eileen Allanmore (née Gaskin, mother), 2–3, 11, 46, 54, 55, 61, 224
Alleyne, Grant (brother), 6–8, 55, *177*
Alleyne, Jacqueline (sister), 8, *177*
Alleyne, Leonora (sister), 8, *177*
Alleyne, Peter (brother), 8, *177*
Alleyne, Sir George, 56, 57; academic achievements and scholarships, 9, 10, 17–18, 19, 38, 46; "Apologia of a Gusanito" farewell address, 94–96; birth of, 3; career overview, ix–xii; childhood and youth, 3–4, 9–13; church influence, 26–27; clinical research, 63–72, 94; courtship and marriage, 32–33, 59, 60, 224–25; as director of PAHO, 125–28, 133–36; Eric Williams Memorial Lecture, 191–92; eulogy for Nettleford, 218; family, role of in development, 4, 26–27; internship, 42–52; music, 224; PAHO acceptance speech, 121, 122–25; PAHO Health Programs Development, 102–4; "Pride in the Product", 207–8; regrets,

259

Index

Alleyne, Sir George (*continued*) 226; retirement consultation, 184; siblings, 177; sources of satisfaction, 226–29; "The Houses that John Built" tribute to Waterlow, 77–79; travelling professorship, 88–89; as UN special envoy on HIV/AIDS, 184–91; as UWI chancellor, 210–16; "Voices of the Pelican", 211–13; "Whither Caribbean Health", 114; WHO director general election campaign, 152–60

Alleyne, Sylvan (née Chen, wife), 46, 58, 61, 93, 121, 180; courtship and marriage to GA, 32–33, 59, 60, 224–25; research work of, 73; social work degrees, 72–73

Alwan, Dr Ala, 200

ammonia, and glucose production, 67–68

Amulree, Lord, 49

Anglican Church: influence of, 26–27; schools established by, 1–2, 10–11

Annamunthodo, Harry, 42, 43

Annan, Kofi, 138, 158, 172, 180; GA as special envoy for HIV/AIDS, 186

Antezana, Dr Fernando, 154

antibiotics, 42

anti-microbial resistance, 202

Antrobus, Ken, 107

Arias, Dr Jaime, 117, 119

Aristotle, *Ethics*, 27, 133–34

Armstrong Memorial Scholarship, 18

Arthur, Owen, 154, 161, 162, *183*, 185, 195, 197

The Ascent of Man (Bronowski), 95–96

Association of Schools of Public Health, 165

Augier, Roy, 207

Barbados: and Alleyne family, 1–9; candidature of GA as director general WHO, 153–60; Carnegie Public Library, 13, 15; chronic disease research centre, 202; clinical teaching in, 92, 93; Freemasons in, 22; and GA as PAHO director, 117–18; Harrison College, 9, 14–18; infant mortality, 5, 10; racial divisions, and cultural elitism, 14, 15, 19, 22–23; riots of 1937, 4–5; social conditions, 4–5

Barbados General Hospital, x, 44–46; nursing staff, 45

Barbados Rediffusion, 9

Barbados Scholarship, 18, 19

Barrett-Sobers, Gloria, 211

Barrow, Dame Nita, 58

Baugh, Eddie, 222

Baugh, Kenneth, 113

Beckles, Sir Hilary, *182*, 208–9, 210, 211; as vice chancellor, 219–20

Bellamy, Carol, 169

Bell-Antoine, Rose-Marie, 189

Bennett, Douglas, 118–19

Bergstrom, Sune, 96

Berkeley, Leonard, 91

Index

Berry, Ronald, 36
Besterman, Harvey, 68
Bethel, Cecil, 30, 32
BHAGs, 163, 164
Black, Sir Douglas, 82
Blackman, Courtney, 27
Blackman, Don, 101-2
Blake, Dr Dorothy, 104, 112, 113
Blake, Evon, 23
Blau, Peter, *Bureaucracy in Modern Society*, 137
Bloomberg, Michael, 204
Boletin Panamericano de Salud, 136
Bolt, Usain, 183
books and literature, 12-13, 15-16
Boston University, 67-68
Bourne, Compton, 195
Bowen, Francis, 22
boxing, 16
Boyd, Dr Philip, 101, 107-8, 115
Bradshaw, Sonny, 224
brain drain, and postgraduate training, 84
Brandling-Bennett, David, 131
Bronowski, Jacob, *The Ascent of Man*, 95-96
Brown, Mr, 36
Brown, Veta, 194, 195
Brown, Vincent, 25
Brundtland, Dr Gro Harlem, 171, 180; as candidate WHO director general, 152-53, 154, 155, 158, 161
Built to Last (Collins), 163
Bunje, Dr Henry, 82
Bureaucracy in Modern Society (Blau), 137

bureaupathology, and corruption, 137
Burton, Carlisle, 15, 108
Byer, Dr Maurice, 44, 62, 63

Caines, John, 113
Canada: and Caribbean Public Health Agency, 115; funding for NCDs, 197; and GA as candidate WHO director general, 156; and PAHO, 105
carbon tetrachloride, and hookworm infection, 75
cardiovascular disease, 87
Caribbean: brain drain, and postgraduate training, 84; health, development and tourism, 167; and health security, 202-4; impact of HIV/AIDS, 184-90; major health problems facing, 194
Caribbean Broadcast Media Partnership on HIV/AIDS (CBMP), 189
Caribbean Business Coalition, 188
Caribbean Community (CARICOM): Commission on Health and Development, 194; cooperation in health initiative, 110-14; and GA as candidate WHO director general, 154, 162; and GA as PAHO director, x, 116, 118; and Global Health Security initiative, 203-4; Liliendaal Resolution, 199; and PAHO, 101, 104, 106-9, 172
Caribbean Consultative Group, 185

261

Index

Caribbean Cooperation in Health initiative, 109, 110–14, 143, 194; financial resource mobilization, 113; ministerial mission, 113; objectives, and project development priorities, 112; project evaluations, 112, 114; "Whither Caribbean Health", 114
Caribbean Development Bank, 195
Caribbean Drug Testing Laboratory, 115
Caribbean Environmental Health Institute, 115
Caribbean Epidemiology Center (CAREC), 108–9; and HIV/AIDS effort, 184–85
Caribbean Food and Nutrition Institute (CFNI), 77, 115
Caribbean Group for Cooperation in Economic Development, 185
Caribbean Health Research Council, 74
Caribbean Public Health Agency, 114–15; and health security, 203–4
CARICOM. *See* Caribbean Community (CARICOM)
Carnegie Public Library, 13, 15
Carrington, Edwin, 196, 206
Carrington, Lawrence, 209
Cartey, Wilfred, 70–71
Castro, Fidel, 94, 170, 179
Catholic University (Maryland), 73
Champagnie, Dunstan, *The Book of the Dead*, 40
champions for change programme, 188
Chen, Carmen, 60

Chen, Sylvan. *See* Alleyne, Sylvan (née Chen, wife)
Chevannes, Barry, 217
chikungunya, 202
childhood mortality: and acute respiratory infections, 103–4; infant mortality, 5, 10
cholera, 98, 109, 139, 169, 227
Chrétien, Jean, 156
chronic diseases, 112
civil rights struggle, x, 29
Clayton, Cecile, 207
Cleveland, Harlan, 135
clinical research: and principles of academia, 95; and technological issues in developing countries, 71–72. *See also* renal function research
Clinton, Hillary, 170
Cochrane, Archie, 49–50
Codrington College (Barbados), 30
Collins, James, *Built to Last*, 163
colonialism: racial divisions, and cultural elitism, 14, 15, 19, 22–23
Commonwealth Caribbean Medical Research Council: as Caribbean Health Research Council, 74; GA as scientific secretary, 73–75
Commonwealth Foundation, and African universities, 86–87
Commonwealth Secretariat, 213
Conference(s) of Health Ministers, 110
conflict management, 45
Cooney, Henry, 107
corruption: and bureaupathology, 137; vote buying, 159

Index

cricket, 16–17
Cropper, Angela, 112, 113
Cruickshank, Eric, 25, 34, 42, 46; University Hospital of the West Indies, 51, 80
Cuba: health indicators, 170; technical cooperation by, 142–43
cultural diversity, 147–48
Cummings, Dr Hugh, 98
Cummings, Rudy, 197

Daniel, Rudolph, 15, 16, 62, 63
DDT, and malaria, 74–75
Demerara Doctor (Giglioli), 75
dengue, 172
Desnoes and Geddes, 91
developmental psychology, and infant malnutrition research, 65
diabetes, 87; and death of Grant Alleyne, 7–8
Dingwall, David, 155, 156
Diouf, Dr Marie-Andre, 105
disease: and illness, distinction between, 33–34; regional immunization programmes, x, 103, 168, 227–28
Douglas, Dr Denzil, 171, 197, 200
Downs, Dr Wilbur, 108
Drayton, Harold, 101–2
Drucker, Peter, 137
Drummond, Don, 224
Dumont, Ivy, 121
Dunn Nutritional Laboratory (Cambridge), 80–83
Duvalier, Dr François, 127–28
Dyer, Dr Halmond, 111

economic development: and health, 191–93; Commission on Macroeconomics and Health, 194
Effectiveness and Efficiency (Cochrane), 50
Eisenberg, Leon, 96
Eliot, T.S., 135
environmental protection, 112
epidemiology, and health situation analysis, 167
Epstein, Dr Eve, 158
equity, and thesis of proportionality, 27
Eric Williams Memorial Lecture, 191–92
Escoffrey, Dr, 31
ethnomedicine, 5
Evans family, 24
evidence-based medicine, 50

The Face of Man (Alleyne), 192
family: role of in development, 26–27; value of, 4
Fellowship of the Royal College of Physicians and Surgeons (Canada), 85
Feng, Dr Paul, 32
Ferdinand, Dr Elizabeth, 157
Ferreira, José Roberto, 100
Figueroa, John, 207
Finlay, Carlos, 98
First Ladies of the Americas meetings, 170
Fitzgerald, Ella, 224
Flores, Hernando, 68
folk medicine, 5
food, and nutrition, 112

Index

Forde, Harold, 44, 47, 225
Forrester, Terrence, 195
Frank, Joe, 16
Fraser, Henry, 69, 222
Freeland, Adolphus, 113
Freemasons, 22
Frenk, Dr Julio, 156, 171
Fukuyama, Francis, 27

Galdo, Magaly, 97
Garrow, John: and Commonwealth Caribbean Medical Research Council, 74; and TMRU, 63, 64
gender inequality: of Caribbean women, 167–68; and HIV/AIDS, 187–88
Getting to Yes (Fisher and Ury), 205
Ghana, Cape Coast and El Mina, 87
Giglioli, Dr George: DDT, and malaria, 74–75
Gittens, Mr, 15
Glaxo Fellowship, 46
global health: and health security, 202–4; politics of, x–xi
Global Health Security initiative, 203–4
global sanitary conferences, 97–98
gluconeogenesis, 67–68
Golding, Bruce, 197
Golding, John, 34; Kendal train crash, 36–37; poliomyelitis epidemic, 35
Gonsalves, Ralph, 198
Gore, Al, 130
Greaves, Stanley, 11
Green, Hamilton, 113

Greene, Dr Eddie, 191, 193, 197, 207
Grenada Boys School, 29
Gutierrez, Ramon Alvarez, 104

Hackett, Christopher, 200
Hagley, Knox, 20, 28, 29–30, 37, 60, *176*
Haiti, and PAHO, 104–5
Hall, Kenneth, *183*
Hall, Marshall, 209, 210–11
Hammond, J.C., 18
Haq, Mahbub ul, 192
Harlem Renaissance, x, 29
Harper, Stephen, 197
Harper, Walter, 31
Harris, Nigel, *182*, *183*, 195, 210, 211; as vice chancellor, 218–19
Harrison College, 9, 14–18
Hassell, Cedric, 38
Hassell, Sir Trevor, 201
Hayes, John, 76
health, and human rights, 170
health equity, xi, 130; horizontal vs vertical equity, 133–34; and liberal democracy, 27; role of the state in, 114; and social justice, 160
Health in the Americas (PAHO), 172
health information as planning tool, 136
health security, and the Caribbean, 202–4
health systems: measurement of, 169; strengthening of, 112, 169
Healthy Caribbean Coalition, 201
Hemispheric Summits of the Americas, 170, 198–99

Index

Hidalgo, Lily, 139, 148
Hill, Aubyn, 215
Himsworth, Sir Harold, 80, 83
HIV/AIDS, 112, 227; antiretroviral therapy, cost of, 185; Barbados conference on, 185–86; and CBMP, 189; champions for change programme, 188; and human rights, 189–90; impact on Caribbean, 184–90; Joint United Nations Programme on HIV/AIDS (UNAIDS), 151; mother-to-child transmission, 168; Pan Caribbean Partnership against HIV/AIDS, 114; stigma and discrimination, 187–90
Ho Ping Kong, Herbert, 65, 90; sickle-cell anaemia research, 69
Holiday, Billie, 29
Holy Trinity Boys School, 1
hookworm infection, and carbon tetrachloride, 75
Hope Foundation: postgraduate training programme, 84, 85
horizontal equity, 134
Hortelano, Paloma, 94
Horwitz, Dr Abraham, 99, 108, 122, 126, 127–28
Hospedales, James, 195, 197, 198
Hospital for Tropical Diseases, 49
Houseman, A.E., 96
Hudson-Phillips, Archie, 20, 24
Hughes, Langston, 29
human development: and health, 191–93; and non-communicable diseases (NCDs), 192–93
human resources development, 112

human rights, and HIV/AIDS, 189–90
Hunte, Keith, 22
Hurricane Gilbert, 206
Hurricane Mitch, 169
Husbands, Sir Clifford, 182
hypertension, 87

Iglesias, Enrique, 164, 192
illness: among elderly, social problem of, 49; and disease, distinction between, 33–34
Imagination Award, 6
infant and child mortality, 5, 10, 168; and acute respiratory infections, 103–4
infant malnutrition research: and carbohydrate metabolism, 69; play, effect of on childhood development, 65; potassium, and body composition, 68–69; protein calorie malnutrition, 86; renal function, and cardiac output, 64–65; at TMRU, x, 62, 63–69
infectious diseases: anti-measles campaign, 114; Caribbean Cooperation in Health initiative, 109, 110–14; and global health security, 202–4; regional immunization programmes, x, 103, 168, 227–28; regional threat of, 98; smallpox, 135; technical cooperation, and PAHO, 139
information: and commodification of knowledge, 221; PAHO use of, 135–36; value of, 172
Inniss, Edson, 19

Index

innovation, triple helix theory of, 221
Inter-American Development Bank, 127, 192; relationship with PAHO, xi; "Shared Agenda for Health in the Americas", 164
international cooperation: technical cooperation vs technical assistance, 140
International Development Research Centre, 213
International Diabetes Federation, 201
International Health Regulations, 203
International Office of Public Health, 139
International Pediatric Association, 70
International Pediatric Conference, 70
International Union against Cancer, 201
International Union of American States, 98
Israel, Elizabeth "Ma Pampo", *181*
Israel, Kathleen, 104

Jamaica: brain drain, and postgraduate training, 84; clinical medicine comparison to Nigeria, 87; Freemasons in, 22; poliomyelitis epidemic, ix, 35; political unrest, 89–90; racial discrimination, 22–23; Tropical Metabolism Research Unit (TMRU), 62, 63–69

James, C.L.R., 39
James, Philip, 197
Jamison, Dean, 194
Jelliffe, Dick, 77
"Jell-O principle", 104
Jemmot, Ralph, *History of Harrison College*, 14
Jha, Prabhat, 197
"Joe's Nitery", 30
Johns Hopkins Bloomberg School of Public Health, 204–5
Johns Hopkins School of Public Health, 86
Joint United Nations Programme on HIV/AIDS (UNAIDS), 151
Jordan, Oscar, 27

Keeling, Ann, 201
Kendal train crash, 36–37
King, Martin Luther, Jr, 27
Kipling, Rudyard, xi, 161
Knouss, Robert, 125, 131
Kodicek, Dr Ernest, 80, 81
Kumanike, Shiriki, 197
Kumate, Dr Jesus, *177*

Lalor, Noelle, 92, *175*
Lancet Commission: future health threats, 202
Latin American and Caribbean Association for Education in Public Health, 165
Laurie, Dr Peter, 116, 120, 153, 157, 161
Leacock, Dr Allyson, 189
League of Nations, 139
Leloir, Luis, 96

Index

Lewis, Sir Arthur, 72, 147, 191
liberal democracy, and global health equity, 27
Liliendaal Resolution, Thirtieth Meeting of Conference of CARICOM Heads of Government, 199
Lim, Bea, 91
Lim, Jim, 91
Ling, James, 30
London, England: Membership of the Royal Colleges of Physicians (MRCP) examination, 45, 46–51
London School of Economics, 72
London School of Hygiene and Tropical Medicine, 79; and *Demerara Doctor* (Giglioli), 75
Londoño, Juan Luis, 119
Longshaw, Ian, 94
Lopez Acuna, Dr Daniel, 164
Lucas, Dr Adetokunbo, 156
lupus erythematosus, 87

Mac Iver, Dr Cecil, 89
Macedo, Dr Carlyle Guerra de, x, 99, 104, 139, *176*; Caribbean Cooperation in Health initiative, 110–11, 113; cross-programmatic planning of, 131; and GA as PAHO director, 116, 121, 128; "Health as a Bridge for Peace", 227–28; as PAHO director emeritus, 121; PAHO directorship, 101–2, 105, 122, 125–26
MacKay, Ian, 31
Madam Rose, 222
Mahler, Dr Halfdan, 103

Mais, Roger, 42
malaria, and DDT, 74–75
malnutrition. *See* infant malnutrition research
Manley, Michael, 89
Manley, Norman, 73
Mann, Jonathan, 151
Manning, Patrick, *183*, 195, 197, 198, 199
Marquez, Dr Patricio, 189
Marshall, Sir Roy, 82, 86
Marshall, Woodville, 27
Massad, Dr Carlos, 120, 121
maternal and child health programmes, 112, 168
Maxwell, Sybil, 6, 8
Mazza, Dr. Alberto, 132
McDonald, Archibald, *182*
McGill University (Canada), 30
McGregor, Sally, 65
McIntyre, Sir Alister, *178*, 194, 208
Medawar, Peter, *Advice to a Young Scientist*, 66, 67
Medical Research Council, 77; Epidemiology Unit, 49
Melkman family, 47
Meltzer, Richard, 85
Membership of the Royal Colleges of Physicians (MRCP) examination, 45, 46–51; limitations of postgraduate examinations, 85–86
memoir, definition of, ix
Miller, Dame Billie, 153, 157, 161
Millott, Norman, xiii, 21–22
Milstein, Cesar, 96
Minott, Owen, 25–26

267

Missoni, Eduardo, 113
Mona, Valley of, 19, 20–21
"Mona Moon", 25, 29
Morehouse School of Medicine (US), 218
Moreno Rojas, Ivan 121
Morgan, Owen, 92, 94
Morrow, Rufus, 85
Munnings, Hal, 102
Munroe, Dr Trevor, 89
Myrtle Bank Hotel, 23

Nakajima, Dr Hiroshi: as director general of WHO, 105, 119–20, 150–52, 153
National Dance Theatre Company, 216
national development: role of health in, xiii
NCD Alliance, 201
nephrology. *See* renal function research
Nettleford, Rex, 40; Chancellor's Medal, acceptance speech, 217–18; as vice chancellor, 208–9, 211, 216–18
Niehaus, Bernardo, 119
Nigeria: clinical medicine comparison to Jamaica, 87
non-communicable diseases (NCDs), 193–202; Commonwealth Heads of Government meeting, 199–202; global health security, 202–4; and government responsibilities, 195; health insurance, Caribbean-wide, 195; "Health of the Region is the Wealth of the Region", 193–94, 199; Hemispheric Summits of the Americas, 198–99; and human development, 192–93; Johns Hopkins Bloomberg School of Public Health, 204–5; Liliendaal Resolution, 199; NCD Alliance, 201; obesity, 194; political support for, 201; Port of Spain Declaration, 197–98, 199, 201; Port of Spain summit, 196–98
nutrition, and food, 112, 168
Nyerere, Julius, 157
Nymn, Glen, 30

Ochoa, Luis Carlos, 102, 104
Ogata, Sadako, 151
Oluwasanmi, Dr, 86
oral health, 169
Organization of American States, 97–98, 119
organizational efficiency, and bureaucracy, 137
organizational management, 136–38; BHAGs, 163; decision-making, 144–46; for-profit vs intergovernmental organizations, 137–38; managing diversity, 146–48
Ovens, Gerald, 34

Pan American Center for Foot and Mouth Disease, 168
Pan American Health and Education Foundation, 127
Pan American Health Organization (PAHO), 96–100; Advisory Committee on Medical Research,

Index

96–97; Area of Health Programs, x; *Boletin Panamericano de Salud*, 136; budgetary funding, 129; and CAREC, 108–9; and the Caribbean, 106–9; Caribbean Cooperation in Health initiative, 110–14; and Caribbean Food and Nutrition Institute, 77; and Caribbean Public Health Agency, 114–15; and CARICOM, x, 101, 104, 106–9; centennial celebrations, 172; cultural diversity, 147–48; decision-making, 144–46; departure of Alleyne, 171–73; Disaster Preparedness programme, 104, 168, 169–70; election of GA as director, 116–25; Environmental Health and Protection programme, 168; essential public health functions, 165–66; and François Duvalier, 127–28; GA as assistant director, 104–9, *176*; GA as director, xi, 128–32, 163–73; GA as director, acceptance speech, 122–25; Health and Human Development Division, 167; "Health as a Bridge for Peace", 227–28; and health equity, 134–36; Health for All goal, 166; *Health in the Americas*, 172; Health Programs Development, 102–4; Health Promotion and Protection Division, 168; and health security, 202–4; immunization programmes, x, 103, 168, 227–28; infectious diseases, regional threat of, 98; Integrated Management of Childhood Illness programme, 103–4; investment in health and environment, 169–70; managing diversity, 146–48; mandate of, 99; maternal and child health programmes, 112, 168; member states, 99, 170–71; mental health programme, 168; organization management, 136–38; organizational development vs re-engineering, 129–31; origin and history of, 97–99; personnel evaluation, 149; politics within, 101–2; programme evaluation, 148–49; and public health, 118; "Public Health in the Americas", 165; publication of scientific information, 136; publications programme, 169; relationship with WHO, 98–99, 128–29, 171; Research Coordination Unit, x, 99–100; "Shared Agenda for Health in the Americas", 164; Special Program for Health Situation Analysis, 136; technical cooperation, 138–44, 166–67, 169; use of information, 135–36; veterinary public health programme, 168; website introduction, 169; Women, Health and Development programme, 104, 167–68; women's position in, 147; works of, 166–71
Pan American Sanitary Bureau, 128

Index

Pan American Sanitary Code (1924), 98, 133, 139
Pan American Sanitary Organization, 99
Pan Caribbean Partnership against HIV/AIDS (PANCAP), 114; establishment of, 185–86
pan-Americanism, xi, 130, 172; health approach of, 134–35; of technical cooperation among countries (TCC), 144
pandemic influenza, and global health security, 202–4
Parboosingh, Dr J., 73
Parnell, Joan, 91
patient care: empathy and hope, 42–43
patient-centred care, 34
Patterson, P.J., 40, 154, 183; on Rex Nettleford, 217
the *Pelican* (student magazine), 38, 40, 224
penicillin, ix
Pereira, Joe, 214
Pérez de Cuellar, Javier, 191–92
Perez-Miravete, Dr, 97
Perkins, Boy, 16
Pico, Luis Argentino, 132
picong, 30
Picou, David, 63, 74, 76, 79
Piot, Peter, 186
Plato, 27
Pogson, Chris, 94
poliomyelitis: eradication of, 114, 135, 168, 227; Jamaican epidemic of, ix, 35; PAHO immunization programme, 103, 168, 227–28

Popper, Karl, 65–66
population health, 166; and health equity, 134–36
Port of Spain Declaration, 197–98, 199, 201
Prefontaine, Norbert, 105
Preston, Aston, 90, 97
proportionality, thesis of, 27
public health: Caribbean Cooperation in Health initiative, 109, 110–14; concept of, 166; and disease prevention, 227–28; essential functions of, xi, 164–66; government role in, 164–66; nutritional problems of, 80, 82; and PAHO, 118
"Public Health in the Americas" (PAHO), 165
Pygmalion effect, 172, 225–26

Quadros, Dr Ciro de, x, 103, 168
Queen's Royal College (Trinidad), 30

racial discrimination, US experience of, 28
racial divisions: and colonial cultural elitism, 14, 15, 19, 22–23
Rafei, Dr Uton Muchtar, 154, 159
Ragbeer, Dr Mohan, 84
Ramadin, Sonny, 198
Ramphal, Sir Shridath, 179, 206–7, 208
Randle, Philip, 94
Ratan, Prem, 46
Reese, Bert, 31
renal function research, 91–92, 94;

and carbohydrate metabolism, 69; and cardiac output, 64–65; electrolyte research, 48–49; gluconeogenesis, 67–68; rat chow, 71. *See also* clinical research
Reneau, Lilian, 104
Roach, Max, 29
Rob, Dr Vincent, 36, 37
Robbins, Fred, 96
Robinson, Leslie, 86
Rockefeller Foundation: and *Demerara Doctor* (Giglioli), 75; and Johns Hopkins School of Hygiene and Public Health, 204; Trinidad Virus Research Laboratory, 108
Rodriguez, Luis Alberto, 200
Roobol, Ann, 68
Roosevelt, Theodore, 135
Root, Elihu, 134–35
Rosenheim, Max, 46, 47, 48, 63, 93, 225; on Dunn Nutritional Laboratory offer, 80, 81, 83
Roses, Dr Mirta, 114–15, 131–32, 144, 197
Ruder Finn, 156

Sachs, Jeffrey, 194
Sadik, Dr Nafis, 154, 155, 159
Sallam, Dr Ismail, 159–60
Samba, Dr Ebrahim, 154, 159
Samms-Knight, Gloria, 40, 206
Sandiford, Erskine, 117
Sankat, Clement, 182
SARS epidemic, 202
Schmunis, Gabriel, 99, 104
Scientific Advisory Committee. *See* Commonwealth Caribbean Medical Research Council
scientific meetings: Chiang Mai, Thailand, 86; International Pediatric Conference, 70
Scullard, George, 68
Sealey, Karen, 104, 200–201; "Whither Caribbean Health", 114
Second Spring (radio programme), 24
Segovia, Miguel, 107
Shalala, Dr Donna, 157, 158
"Shared Agenda for Health in the Americas", 164
sickle-cell anaemia research, 69
Sillink, Martin, 201
Simmons, Peter, 154–55
Simmons McDonald, Hazel, 182
Sir Arthur Sims Commonwealth Travelling Professorship, 88–89
Sloan, Alfred P., 94
Smith, Adam, *The Wealth of Nations*, 193
Smith, Aurie, 27
Smith, Douglas, 19
Smith, Sir Frederick, 27
Smith, Vernon, 27
Soberon, Dr Guillermo, 105
Sommer, Al, 204
Soper, Dr Fred, 99, 172
Sotelo, Juan Manuel, 116, 118, 120, 139, 143
south-south cooperation, 143
Spence, Leslie, 108
Spinacci, Sergio, 194
sports, 16–17
Springer, Sir Hugh, 81

SS Hope, 84
St Margaret's Boys School, 10–11
St Martin's Boys School, 12
Standard, Kenneth, 46, 47
Stanford, Lloyd, 40
Steiner, Achim, 193
stigma and discrimination of HIV/AIDS, 187–90
Street, Sam, 37
Stuart, Dr Ken, 37, 51
Stuart, Freundel, 189–90
study, discipline of, 16, 27

Taitt, Branford, 117, 157–58
Taylor, Carl, 86, 204
technical cooperation, 138–44, 169; strategic approaches of, 141; triangular cooperation, 143; vs technical assistance, 140
technical cooperation among countries (TCC), 142–44
technical cooperation among developing countries (TCDC), 141–42; as south-south cooperation, 143
Tejada, Dr David, 101
Teruel, Jose, 101
Thomas, Ewart, 206
Thompson, Dudley, 89
Thompson, Elizabeth (Liz), 120, 153, 157, 161
tobacco controls, 171, 197
Treaty of Chaguaramas, 110
triangular cooperation, 143
Trinidad and Tobago: clinical teaching in, 92, 93
Trinidad Virus Research Laboratory, 108

tropical diseases: Hospital for Tropical Diseases, 49
Tropical Metabolism Research Unit (TMRU): infant malnutrition research, x, 62, 63–69, 174; role in development of young scientists, 69; self-experimentation, culture of, 69–70
Truman, Harry, 140
Tuberculosis and Lung Association, 201
Tudor, Cameron, 15

UK Medical Research Council, 80
UNAIDS, 151; GA as special envoy for Caribbean, 186–90
United Fruit Company, 23
United Nations: corruption within election process, xi; Economic and Social Council, 200; Helms/Biden legislation (US), 152; international cooperation, need for, 139–40, 142; Joint United Nations Programme on HIV/AIDS (UNAIDS), 151; Political Declaration on NCDs, 201
United Nations Children's Fund (UNICEF), 111, 169–70
United States: New York City visits, 28–29, 51–52; and PAHO directorship, 118–19; West Indian experience of, 28–29
University College Hospital of the West Indies, 31–38
University College London, x, 46
University College of the West Indies (UCWI): clinical medicine, 32–34; extramural teaching and practice,

Index

34, 35–37; first year medicine, 28–29; football team, 57; freedom vs licence, 23–24; Guild Council, 25; Mona Campus, early years, 20–22; nursing students, 32; the *Pelican*, 38, 40, 224; preclinical medicine, 29–32; relationship between staff and students, 21–22, 23–26; student years, 20–27; tobacco and smoking, 24, 56; University of London affiliation, 38; and West Indian consciousness, 39–41; and West Indian nationalism, 19–20

University Hospital of the West Indies: academic physicians vs private practice, 90–91; annex construction funding, 91; nephrology clinic, 80; physicians as generalists, 90; postgraduate training programme, 84–86; as University College Hospital of the West Indies, 31–38

University of Bristol, 94

University of Canterbury, 94

University of Granada (Spain), 94

University of Guyana, 86

University of Ibadan, 87

University of Ife, 86

University of London: affiliation with UCWI, 38

University of the West Indies, x; alumni as ambassadors, 221–22; "Apologia of a Gusanito" farewell address, 94–96; Caribbean Cooperation in Health initiative, 110–14; chancellor, role and responsibilities of, 209–10; enrolment levels, xi, 220; essential roles of university, 220–21; fiftieth birthday celebration, 207–8; GA as chancellor, xi, 210–16; GA as professor of medicine, 83–92; Gathering of the Graduates, 207; governance of, 213–15; government funding, 221; graduation ceremonies, 220–23; Guild of Graduates, 215–16; honorary graduates, 222; "non-campus countries" as Open Campus, 214, 219; Pelican Awards, 216; personal attention to graduates, 222; postgraduate training and examination, 84, 85–86; quality of graduates, 96; School for Graduate studies, 214; Special Convocation, 206–7; specialist qualification certification, 84–86; strategic planning, 219; transformation of governance structure, xi; Trinidad Virus Research Laboratory, 108; Tropical Metabolism Research Unit (TMRU), x; UWI Alumni Association, 215–16; UWI Medical Alumni Association, 206; valedictorian addresses, 222–23; vice chancellor selection, 210–11; vice chancellors, 216–20

University of the West Indies, St Augustine: Health Economics Unit, 193

University of Toronto: postgraduate training programme, 85

Index

Uton, Dr *See* Rafei, Dr Uton Muchtar

Valentine, Alfred, 198
Vaughan, Sarah, 224
vertical equity, 134
veterinary public health programme, 168
violence, health consequences of, 194
Virtual Health Library of the Americas, 172

Walcott, Derek, 25
Walcott, Dr Jerome, 196
Waldron, Errol, 74
Ward, Eugene, 80
Ward, Frank, 16
Washington, George, 78
Waterlow, John C., x, 38, 80, *175*, 225–26; Advisory Committee on Medical Research (PAHO), 96; Commonwealth Caribbean Medical Research Council, 73, 74; magnanimity of, 76–79; "The Houses that John Built" tribute, 77–79; and TMRU, 62, 63, 65
Webster, Dr Rudi, 117, 118
Weinstock, Herman 121
Weisbrod, Burton, 191
Weiss, Carol, 148
Welch, William, 204
Weller, Tom, 96
West Indian consciousness: and colonial cultural elitism, 19–20; development of, 39–41; role of media in, 40; of UWI graduates, 222–23
West Indies Federation, ix, 40–41, 73
Williams, Eric, 39
Wilson, Dr Ronald, 50–51
Wilson, Wendell, 69
W.K. Kellogg Foundation, 128
women: and gender discrimination, 167–68; and HIV/AIDS, 187–88; marginalization of health, 114; maternal and child health programmes, 168; promotion of within PAHO, 147
Women, Health and Development programme (PAHO), 104, 167–68
Wooding, Sir Hugh, 211
World Bank: Caribbean HIV/AIDS funding, 189; recognition of HIV/AIDS, 185; relationship with PAHO, xi; "Shared Agenda for Health in the Americas", 164
World Development Report on Investing in Health, 194–95
World Health Assembly, 119, 154–55, 201
World Health Organization (WHO): call for reform, 151–52; Caribbean Cooperation in Health initiative, 110–14; director general campaign, x–xi, 152–60; director general election, 160–62; and health security, 203–4; Helms/Biden legislation

(US), 152; Commission on Macroeconomics and Health, 194; Nakajima as director, 105, 119–20, 150–52, 153; relationship with PAHO, 98–99, 128–29, 171, *178*; secret balloting, and vote buying, 159; and technical cooperation, 140, 143; Tropical Disease Research Programme, 97

World Heart Federation, 201
Wynter, Hugh, 91, *175*

yellow fever, 98, 139
Young, Baroness, 113

zika virus, 202

CPSIA information can be obtained
at www.ICGtesting.com
Printed in the USA
LVHW090148031019
632980LV00001B/84/P